Mind Your Own Back

Ancient Wisdom to Heal Your Back

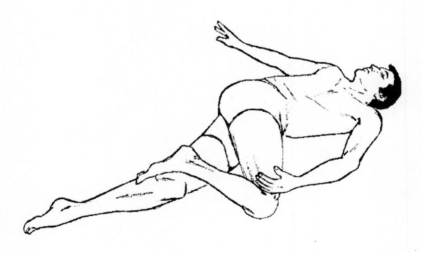

Steve Timm

Revised Edition 2010

With special thanks to the many enthusiastic practitioners of the *Mind Your Own Back* technique.

"*Mind Your Own Back*," by Steve Timm. ISBN 978-1-907547-00-3.

Cover design and illustrations by Steve Timm.

Published 2010 by Creative Productions, 9 Longford Terrace, Monkstown, Co. Dublin, IRELAND 01 2845742

"*The ancient Indian healing traditions of Yoga and Ayurveda are now globally popular. It is deeply satisfying to witness their revival.*

In Mind Your Own Back, Steve Timm clearly and succinctly describes the mechanics of the spine. He then uses this description to help readers align their awareness, feelings, insights, and thinking while performing his unique "pelvis setting" postures. This integration of mind and body stimulates realignment. Steve's direction in this book will empower you to achieve better posture and a healthier structure."

Dr. Donn Brennan, MB. BCh. BAO. MRCGP. MSc. Ayu. Founding President of the UK Ayurvedic Practitioners Association. (UKAPA).

☉☉☉

Great results have been reported after only one or two sessions of Steve Timm's Mind Your Own Back technique. The trend is very encouraging. Many people coming for rejuvenation to our Ayurveda Clinic in Hyderabad, India have reported great benefits from the MYOBack techniques. The technique is excellent when it is integrated with panchakarma procedures. Most people mention fast progress as balance is obtained from the correct setting of the pelvis. More flexibility and easy flow of movements makes people feel and stand taller as walking becomes joyful. We have seen extraordinary recoveries even from a totally collapsed sacrum lumbar joint that surgeons were planning to operate and fuse.

Most people like to be able to understand and to be in control of their own health.

Vaidya Dr. A. V. Raju

Table of contents

Acknowledgments

I wish to offer this book to all the great wise men and teachers who have blessed my life. They gave me the means to cognize everything I need to know to enjoy good health and happiness, and to make progress in my personal evolution, as well as the ability to pass knowledge on to others in need of self-healing. I am also deeply indebted to my mother and those wise old neighbors from my childhood.

I also wish to acknowledge the great contribution that so many happy practitioners of the *Mind Your Own Back* technique have made in an effort to update and improve this Revised Edition of the *Mind Your Own Back* book.

The tradition of Ayurvedic doctors and Vaidyas of India provided me great help and wisdom in fine fine-tuning the *MYOBack* technique. Many thanks to the Raju's family and their tradition of grate Vaidyas for sharing their wealth of Vedic knowledge.

In addition, Dr. Abraham Maslow's clear vision helped me understand the inner workings of the human mind and the natural desire to achieve the highest state of awareness, or "peak experience," that is the benchmark for all successful people. According to Maslow, when this state of pure creative consciousness or Being is attained, any work performed contains a more complete knowledge. Hopefully this book achieves this quality of wholeness.

I give especially warm thanks to His Holiness Maharishi Mahesh Yogi for his simple but most effective Transcendental Meditation technique which gave me the means to contact Being and thereby achieve Maslow's ideal state of consciousness to fulfill my potential.

With deepest gratitude to my source of creativity and inspiration, the great Gurus, Masters and Shankaracharyas who, throughout time, have kept the light of Vedic wisdom shining for all generations to come. I would like to place this work at the Lotus Feet of Shri Guru Deva Bhagwan Swami Brahmananda Saraswati, Shankaracharya of Jyotir Math, Himalayas. May his glorious blessings come to all those who wish to enjoy the glories of life, both mundane and Divine.

All glory to Guru Dev
and the Holy Tradition of Vedic Masters.

Dedication

This book is intended for those who would like to explore new realities in their lives, and who are open to all possibilities. May bliss, happiness and total support of Natural Law be your new reality.

Introduction

When I was a child I felt like a superman. I grew up tall and strong. Water sports were my favorite, especially rowing and swimming in the rivers and lakes surrounding my family home in the South of Chile. I used my physical strength without any concern for (or even awareness of) the damage I might be doing to my body. Like many others fortunate to be born with good health, I was both ignorant and arrogant in my attitude towards maintaining it. When we are young, we can't ever imagine not having a vital physiology and a strong and flexible back. We feel immortal. We are gods. Nothing can ever harm us. We ignore the signs and warnings our bodies telegraph to us. We override pain; push our muscles, ligaments and joints beyond their natural capacity. Consequently we accumulate wear and tear, strain after strain, layer after layer of exertion, until one day we realize things don't seem to work quite the way they used to.

In my case everything began to fall apart in 1974 when an accident at work, while carrying a heavy piece of a main frame computer, left me frozen with pain and flat on my back in bed, unable to move for a whole month. The agony was so immediate and overwhelming I had no choice but to give myself over to medical practitioners to perform their expected miracles and take away my pain. For the first time I was no longer in charge of my life but dependent on others. It was a huge blow to my ego. In matters of strength and health, I had always prided myself on my self-sufficiency and suddenly it was gone.

Eventually I recovered enough from my injury to get out of bed and resume my life. I had no idea of the real damage done to my back and did none of the things necessary to keep it strong and healthy. Over the next fifteen years I suffered all kinds of damage to my back, all of which I ignored in the same way. By 1991 X-ray examinations and an MRI revealed not only had I seriously sprained my back, but also the years of physical abuse and neglect had resulted in serious degeneration of the vertebrae. My spine, the foundation of my bodily strength, was literally crumbling away. After numerous treatments by osteopaths, chiropractors and physical therapists, I was told nothing more could be done. I would have to live in pain for the rest of my life. One specialist told me the only solution was to "get a new body"! I was disabled, cast out by the medical system, another insurance statistic. I'd hit my lowest point of misery and suffering.

In retrospect this was a blessing. Nobody was going to miraculously cure me, so I was forced back onto my own resources. If I wanted to be pain free, strong and flexible ever again, it was up to me, and only me. It was a turning point both physically and spiritually.

Phoenix from the Ashes

We all have a tremendous potential to heal ourselves. We lose sight of how much power we have within us. All that is required is the ability to trust our own intelligence and to listen to the quiet voice that whispers to us in our deepest moments of inner peace and silence.

When I heard there was no hope for a cure, I came to the realization that I would have to live the rest of my life in pain or find the miracle that would cure my condition.

I had a natural inclination to go into silence to refresh myself. In the early 1970's I had attended a number of personal development courses at work which had been used by NASA to prepare astronauts for the first landings on the Moon. It was there I first came across the work of pioneering psychologist Abraham Maslow. I found his insights into the workings of the mind extremely enlightening and from them developed a keen interest in reaching what Maslow called "Peak Experience," which he felt was the highest level of human experience and which was common to all the most creative and successful people. Inspired by this goal, I developed my own system of meditation that led me to deeper and deeper levels of silence and peace.

Following that inner journey came the response I was looking for. There were no clear verbal messages or ideas, just faint impulses to do this or try that. The healing techniques I eventually developed and that are offered to you in the following chapters came to me not as intellectual deduction but rather as whispers of intuition. I began an intimate dialog with my body at the faintest level of feeling. It was a condition of total surrender and without any expectation. I was neither trying to understand the process nor was I attempting to "heal" myself. I knew I was on the right track when I began to experience some bliss and happiness emerging from beneath the pain and suffering. It didn't happen overnight but a little bit at a time, I began to be stronger. Eventually the day came when I realized all the pain was gone. It wasn't until after the healing had taken place that I retraced my steps of recovery and began to understand intellectually the mechanics of the process that healed me.

In the western world, many find it difficult to understand or trust instinctive or intuitive knowledge. The rationale of science and proof by objective experiment is the golden rule. But the truth is that human beings have an infinite potential of knowledge deep within if only we can learn how to access it. This kind of knowledge exists in virtual or potential form and only emerges as subtle sense and intuition. It is not something you can necessarily prove objectively but you can "know" it with certainty.

In 1989 I learned the Transcendental Meditation (TM) technique; a simple procedure that allows one to access Being, the deepest, most silent level of human consciousness in the most systematic way. When I practiced this meditation I found myself experiencing a most profound and joyful bliss, a state of inner being where I was completely at peace and free from the trials and tribulations of everyday life. I was also completely without pain.

According to the literature on the TM technique, the quietest state of the mind is a field of infinite creativity from which emerges all possible knowledge. Transcending the superficial thinking level of the mind allows us to gain access to this knowledge. Maslow's description of Peak Experience seemed to match the state of mind I experienced during TM. I was able to get first hand experience of the huge potential of intelligence that resides deep within the mind and this helped me both verify and understand the power and validity of intuitive knowledge.

The TM technique comes from a very ancient tradition of knowledge called the Vedic tradition, which has been passed on from generation to generation since time immemorial. According to this tradition, all knowledge (Veda) emerges directly from this state of inner Being, which is the origin of all creative intelligence and is available to anyone who can reach that refined state of awareness. All that is required to access this field of "all possibilities" is the ability to transcend our mental and physical awareness. "Established in Being, perform action" is one of the key tenets in the Bhagavad-Gita, the "handbook" of Vedic wisdom.

The Vedic tradition contains practical knowledge to cover all areas of life, from individual health and education (including higher states of consciousness), to agriculture, architecture and government. All these different approaches have a common foundation, which is to align life with the fundamental laws of nature that govern the entire universe. If myriads of stars and galaxies can be organized efficiently and without apparent effort, why not individual health and welfare? Ayurveda (the science of life) is the branch of Vedic Science dealing with health. Ayurveda regards the human mind and body not as separate entities but as one whole, the mind being nothing more than the subtle aspect of the body. This approach allows a much more comprehensive and effective strategy for creating perfect health.

What emerged intuitively as a cure for my chronic back problems, coming as it did from a very holistic state of awareness, included approaches to heal more than just the physical injuries to my spine. They also include practical measures to keep both the mind and body healthy. Back problems do not come just from physical injuries. They are also due to the accumulation of mental and physical stress resulting from poor lifestyle choices, living as it were outside of or in contradiction to the laws of nature that normally uphold good health. If we want to maintain good back health, we have to do more than be careful how we lift heavy objects, though of course that is important.

While traveling in India recently I was fortunate to meet with a number of expert Ayurvedic doctors and Vaidyas. With their help, I was not only able to verify a number of my intuitions about maintaining a healthy back but also received a lot of additional expert advice which is included in this book.

From Student to Teacher

I never expected to use my intuitive discoveries to heal anyone but myself, but shortly after my back was restored to full functioning, my youngest daughter, Cecilia, was involved in a bad car accident in which she ruptured three discs at the base of her spine and sustained injuries to the thoracic (thorax) and cervical (neck) region of the vertebral column. For nearly five years she was in agony. None of the standard treatments worked even though she consulted with the top specialists in Australia, where we were living at the time. Much to my frustration, she wasn't at all interested in hearing my advice on how to treat her injuries.

Cecilia's condition continued to deteriorate to the point where normal painkillers were useless and she needed heavy medication to survive. Eventually she needed sixty milligrams of slow release morphine every day. Her life fell apart. Not only was her career gone and most of her savings, but she lost touch with many of her friends. She had a constant battle with the insurance company to prove her claim. (People with back injuries don't get much compensation in Australia, in the first place.)

Litigation and insurance claims can be a real drain and interfere with the process of healing because the desire to get compensation or to force the other party to accept responsibility for the incident creates contradictory forces in the psychology. One part of you wants to focus on healing while the other wants to demonstrate how bad the condition is so you can receive your rightful compensation. This can be a drag on healing.

When, in desperation, Cecilia finally decided to try *MYOBack*, she agreed to my request to seek a fast out-of-court settlement with the insurance company so she could concentrate on healing. Some members of the family didn't agree as they felt Cecilia was owed a lot for her injuries and they wanted to get even with those who had caused them, but Cecilia was tired of the insurance warfare.

Dropping the internal conflicts over getting a settlement allowed her to focus on getting better.

What she was doing was practicing the art of "surrendering," which is very important in the healing process. It requires accepting that there are no mistakes in life. If something happens to us, it is usually for a good reason. In reality, everything happens exactly the way it should according to the laws of cause and effect. Ultimately we create our own universe. What we experience in the present is due to our actions in the past. What we will experience in the future will be based on what we do today. It is the inexorable law of cause and effect, more often known these days as karma, a term originating from the Vedic tradition. Ayurveda aims at keeping the whole of our life in balance in order that no harm is done to us or to others.

We all have our own "currency" in life to spend the way we choose. Contrary to many people's belief it is not the accumulation of dollars and cents that matters but rather how and where we allocate our precious time and energy. God gives everybody the same twenty-four hours a day to make good use of or to waste, as we wish. Especially when we are sick, rather than wasting valuable resources feeling bad about ourselves or blaming others for our problems, that time and energy can be more usefully used to get whole again.

It was important to attend to Cecilia's body–mind relationship before proceeding to fix the physical ailment. I suggested she seek her body's consent to allow the healing to take place, and, most importantly, to ask for a clear signal of approval once the process was begun. I explained to her that with this treatment she was to listen to her body and treat it with love and respect. Most importantly, she was going to be the one taking responsibility for her own healing. Five or ten minutes after the initial session, the answer from her body came back loud and clear. She was lying on the couch resting after treatment, when a wave of bliss and energy swept through her body and into her legs. This convinced her to continue with the program.

A month later, when she visited her rheumatologist, he was amazed by her progress. He was immediately able to cut her pain medications in half.

MYOBack didn't fix all of Cecilia's problems.

A chronic pain that persisted for many years will cause damage to the nervous system and there will still be pain even if the cause of pain was removed. Cecilia had to go through pain management and battle the addiction caused by the drugs.

After a long battle Cecilia made impressive recovery thanks to her tenacity and determination

Within a year, Cecilia was feeling much stronger and she was able to go back to swim and work out in the gym once more. Interviewed in the Australian magazine *Cleo* at the successful outcome of her treatment, she was able to say, "I did it my way."

Birth of the *MYOBack* Technique.

My daughter's miraculous recovery convinced me God had given me a truly precious gift that needed be shared with others. I formulated everything I learned into a program designed to enable everyone to maintain a healthy back. I decided to call it the *Mind Your Own Back* (*MYOBack*) technique, because it's a program that can be largely implemented on your own.

The book has two purposes. For those who are physically in good shape and have a good healthy back, it is intended to provide you with the knowledge to maintain your back in good condition, keeping it flexible and strong, thus allowing the free flow of nervous energy along the spine. Therefore achieving what the great yogis aspire to achieve for the purpose of evolution. For those of you who are recovering from back injuries or damage to the spine, it is intended to help in the rehabilitation from your injuries and the prevention of further damage. Self-sufficiency in back care is the goal.

How to Learn the *Mind Your Own Back* technique.

Learning *Mind Your Own Back* is easy as A B C.

The *MYOBack* technique is very easy to learn. It involves coordination of mind body and prana (breathing).

Just as in this book you will simply need to follow the simple A B C steps to get it right. It is highly recommended to observe the sequence as there is mental preparation to do before the first practice session. This is important if you want to get good results. Remember that you are in control and it is your duty to *Mind Your Own Back.*

A – Step 1. Understanding your Spine. This is described in Chapter 1 of this book and it is the basis for your mental preparation.

Even if you have already read this book you should still review the initial part of the training DVD set.

This will give you an insight in the working of the spine to help you to understand its needs and what to do to keep it healthy.

B – Step 2. Initial learning of the *Mind Your Own Back* technique.

The actual practice of the first *MYOBack* routine should only be performed after a clear understanding of the Spine and its needs.

It is highly advised to do the full *MYOBack* routine "*in your mind first*" in order to complete the mental preparation before the first practice session.

C – Step 3. The first practice comes after the initial preparation thus allowing the mind to be with the different parts of the spine and body that you are working on. You can then be totally relaxed and focus on the body and the application of the *MYOBack* technique without any mental doubt or concern.

Additional yoga asanas are also included in this book as well as in the practice DVD's.

Who should you learn *Mind Your Own Back from.*

You should learn from a proper legitimate source.

It is said that bad backs are products of bad past karma. People that believe or understand karma will avoid incurring into bad karma by avoiding unlawful use of this or any other knowledge or technique.

If an illegal copy of the book or DVD is what awakened the interest to learn *MYOBack*, it is highly advisable to get a legitimate legal copy to enjoy the full benefits of this powerful technique. You need an easy and relax mind free of any guilt or concern.

The laws of Karma are very much the same as the laws of cause and effect. Action and reaction.

Learning from the source.

Old wisdom tells us that the best way to learn anything is from the very source of knowledge. The next best option would be to learn from a certified trained *MYOBack* professional in order of finding the most advisable method of learning and applying the exercises of the *MYOBack* technique.

This book is designed for general back health to provide as much information as possible on the *MYOBack* technique. What is in the book is considered safe for the general public to know without the assistance of a trained professional.

Learning from DVD's.

As an alternative to learning from a professional trainer DVD's are available for visual assistance as well as spoken instructions during learning. However it is highly recommended to read the *Mind Your Own Back* book before the first learning practice.

Learning from DVD's will be the closest thing to learning from the source with the only exception being that there will be no professional trainer observing your practice and making any necessary corrections.

The DVD's are recommended for people to use in the practices following direct learning from a trained professional. It will help to make sure the practice is kept in its original form and intention. It is said that humans need to have 190 repetitions to learn something new and if you are a genius you only need 150 repetitions. So it is highly suggested to use the DVD's for all the learning period.

It is recommended keeping the learning DVD's after learning, as they may become handy in case of some back injury or back problem.

Learning from this book.

If applied with caution the instructions on this book should be a safe way for you to learn a simple version of the *MYOBack* technique.

Caution is advised with complex or chronic back conditions as they may require consultation with a medical expert or a trained *MYOBack* professional. In the case of treating chronic back conditions, there are specialized aspects to the *MYOBack* technique that cannot be included in this book as they require individual application under trained supervision. However if your case is simple, I will strongly recommend the knowledge and exercises exposed in this book combined with the instructional DVD's.

Watch the web page: www.mindyourownback.com or www.myoback.com and look for information about DVD's and other *MYOBack* products as they become available. The intention is to make you self-sufficient in your back care for the future.

For further information on *MYOBack* products and services please refer to the above mentioned Internet website where you can find the location and availability of certified *MYOBack* experts trained in the *MYOBack* technique as well as finding about Videos, DVD's and other *MYOBack* products as they become available.

So this is my sincere offering to you, with gratitude to those great masters and teachers who helped me uncover and adapt this advance yoga or *MYOBack* technique to make it easy for average people to benefit. I hope this knowledge helps you as it did me and the many others to whom I have since taught this simple but very powerful technique.

Wishing you a strong and healthy spine.

Steve Timm, 12 January 2007

Disclaimer

Anyone with a history of serious birth malformations in the spine, degeneration of the spine, scoliosis, collapsed discs or who has had any kind of surgery to the spine, or those with a history of mental instability should seek advice from a medical professional before attempting to practice the methods and techniques described in this book.

No promises are made that the *MYOBack* technique will help or cure any particular case of back problem or injury. Since *MYOBack* is a self applied technique the stories mentioned in the book are personal achievements.

PART I
UNDERSTANDING THE PROBLEM

Chapter 1
Understanding your Spine

The human vertebral column is a beautiful example of the logic and precision of natural intelligence. Constructed from a complex interaction of bone, muscle, nerves and other soft tissue, it provides the essential framework for the functioning of your whole body. The main function of the vertebral column is to provide a flexible protected channel for the spinal cord to run through its length bringing nerve supply and nerve connections to the entire body. Ancient yogis understood the importance of maintaining a flexible and healthy spine not only for ongoing health and vitality but also for spiritual growth. They devised a simple series of exercises, lifestyle choices and dietary programs designed to prevent back problems and maintain good posture and a healthy spine. These are the foundation of the *MYOBack* program.

With today's world and stressful lifestyle, back related health problems are now becoming pandemic and responsible for much pain, suffering and lost work and recreation time. In almost all cases, if attended to in a timely fashion, back problems can be treated easily and future problems prevented by using this ancient Vedic wisdom. Painful and dangerous surgery, which may be necessary when back problems become very serious, can also be avoided.

Before describing the Vedic approach to treating back problems, let's first gain an understanding of the spine, how it is constructed and why and where back problems arise in the first place.

The origins and evolution of the spine

Vertebral columns or spines appear in the most primitive forms of life. Prehistoric fish had a flexible column of cartilage running through the center of their bodies, which provided the structural anchor for the powerful muscles required to either catch their prey or escape from predators.

When these sea creatures left the ocean and evolved into reptiles, big modifications were necessary to the original design of the spine. In order to deal with the powerful force of gravity that came into play standing up on solid ground, the spinal column moved away from the center of the body and vertebrae were formed of bone instead of cartilage matter. A different combination of facet joints, ligaments and muscles was needed to hold the structure together, but the basic principles remained the same.

The vertebral column had to be flexible in order to bend and twist in all directions and this required a coordinated symphony of muscles and ligaments in the interconnectedness between the different parts. That is why flexing and exercise is essential to keeping the spine healthy. External muscles such as those in the abdomen were also developed to maintain the internal strength to support the expansion or decompression of the discs, an important function of a healthy back. The spine also housed and protected the web of nerves carrying the flow of energy throughout the body.

The human spine—our own balancing act.

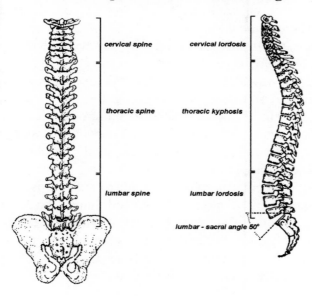

cervical spine   cervical lordosis

thoracic spine   thoracic kyphosis

lumbar spine   lumbar lordosis

lumbar - sacral angle 50°

Fig. 1. The vertebral column.

Once the spine became vertical, a number of problems arose. The human spine consists of twenty-four moving vertebrae, which are stacked on top of each other arising from the "foundation stone" in the sacrum and pelvis. In order to stay balanced, the segments of the spine are arched forward and backward from the central line of gravity in three gentle curves like a cobra, enchanted by the sound of a flute, rising gracefully from a basket. The hollow curve in the lower back is called the *lumbar lordosis (curve)*.

Above this is the *thoracic hump,* a longer, gentler curve in the opposite direction in the thoracic region, leading into the curve in the neck area called the *cervical lordosis (curve)*. In order to maintain this curvaceous balancing act, the sacrum-lumbar joint had to be set at an angle of fifty degrees. Prolonged sitting at our desks or on the sofa watching TV can diminish this lumbar curve, tipping the pelvis backwards and throwing out the balance of the whole spine.

The sacrum-pelvis with its fifty-degree angle tilt at the base of the spine is the foundation of the building. If strong and properly positioned, this foundation ensures proper functionality of the spine, including the right curves for shock absorption and correct distribution of body weight throughout the front and back components of the spine. For example, the slight bowing forward in the lumbar region helps absorb impact while walking.

The loss of the correct lumbar curve is usually accompanied by a more pronounced hunch back in the thoracic region and a sharp backward turn of the neck, as the body struggles to maintain its balance against gravity. Problems can then manifest in different parts of the spine, especially if there are areas of weakness.

The vertebrae

The vertebrae are the individual segments of the spine. In between the vertebrae are discs, which act as flexible links and shock absorbers.

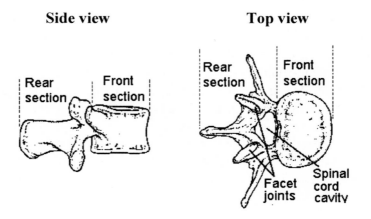

Fig. 2. A vertebra.

The front of the vertebra is shaped like a drum, which is specifically designed for stacking one on top of the other and bearing most of the weight. The back contains the facet joints that interlock the spinal segments together so they stay in place, plus some drumstick pieces of bone for the ligaments and muscles to attach to. It also includes a protective cavity for the delicate spinal cord to run through.

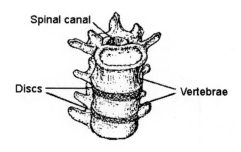

Fig. 3. Vertebrae and discs.

The vertebrae are not solid, but instead made of bone, which is porous and honeycomb-like in consistency and full of blood under pressure. This allows them to act like hydraulic drums, helping to absorb impact. The front section also provides the fluids and nutrients that are fed into the discs by the alternation of compression and decompression as we move the back.

The Discs

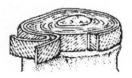

Fig. 4. The disc.

The discs between the vertebrae keep the front section of the vertebrae from rubbing against each other while providing a well-cushioned spacer that allows the joint to be flexible and able to absorb impact. The center of the disc is filled with a mucous substance with a very high fluid absorption and retention capacity. This mucous fluid is held at the center of the disc by a dozen thin layers of diagonally alternating strong fibrous material with a consistency and structure similar to the layers of rubber in a radial car tire.

Fluids and nutrients feeding the discs

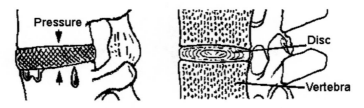

Fig. 5. The flow of nutrients.

The discs have no blood supply of their own and depend completely on the fluids and nutrients fed to them by the vertebrae. When the compression is released the disc "breathes in" to absorb nutrients, and, under pressure, "breathes out" to release toxic waste. Like all natural systems, the spine requires alternate rest and activity to stay healthy. If subject to sustained pressure for long periods, the discs will lose fluid and slowly dry up, and the fibrous layers will bulge outwards. The joints become floppy and unstable like car tires without sufficient air. But the discs will also bounce back quickly when given the opportunity to do so during rest or stretching.

Long hours sitting down without much movement makes the discs go low on fluids, creating stiffness and making it painful to stand up and stretch. At the end of the day you will be shorter than you were in the morning due to the drying out and shrinking of the discs. Normally discs will recover their fluid content during rest at night but an imbalance of activity over rest will create problems long term. A little bit of attention to flexing and exercising the spine on a regular basis goes a long way in maintaining a youthful and healthy spine.

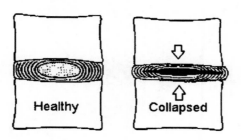

Fig. 6. Internal ruptures can occur in an accident.

During an accident, discs can be ruptured or damaged. Muscle spasms may then hold the damaged joint tight for a long time. A damaged disc can't swell and deflate and will be less able to absorb impact (Figure 6.). In the worse case scenario, the disc will burst and leak fluid causing severe irritation to the nerves located immediately outside the discs. This is what happened to my daughter Cecilia after her car accident, causing severe inflammation in the low lumbar region and triggering more muscle spasms that aggravated the problem. Before healing could begin, the ruptured disc walls needed a chance to close up and repair themselves.

The base of the spine receives the maximum weight load and therefore the lower discs tend to suffer maximum compression and fluid loss. This situation is even worse at the very first joint (L5/S1) where the required fifty-degrees angle makes it even more difficult for the joint to recover from damage or compression.

The butterfly in you.

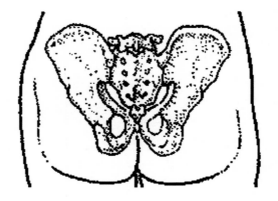

Fig. 7. The butterfly.

The key component that holds the spine is shaped like a butterfly. In India, it is sometimes thought of as the elephant god Ganesh holding up the spine with his immense strength. Even though the components of the sacrum-lumbar region are substantial in size, there is also a complex network of nerves that can get easily trapped by the large bone structures. Any misalignments or changes at the sacrum-lumbar area will affect the rest of the spine.

Fig. 7 shows the sacrum and pelvis as seen from behind. The sacrum is the central bone and it has eight holes through which eight major nerves pass that serve crucial parts of the physiology. Linked on both sides of the sacrum are the two halves of the pelvis. At the lowest part of the pelvis we have what are called the *sitting bones.*

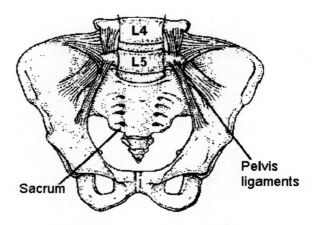

Fig. 8. Front of the sacrum, pelvis and links.

The sacrum and pelvis are linked to the L5 and L4 vertebra by a network of strong internal as well as external muscles and ligaments that constitute the key components in the foundation of the human spine. Keeping the correct balance of right and left plus the proper length of these ligaments is key to keeping the pelvis seated at the correct angle and position.

The sacrum-lumbar region is so delicate that surgery is highly complicated and dangerous and I believe is best avoided if at all possible. Inserting metal plates and pins or artificially fusing vertebrae may offer short-term solutions but generally can lead to serious long-term problems.

The inter-vertebral muscles

Inter-vertebral muscles, often called ligaments, are plaited along the vertebrae holding them all together in a well-balanced way (Fig. 9).

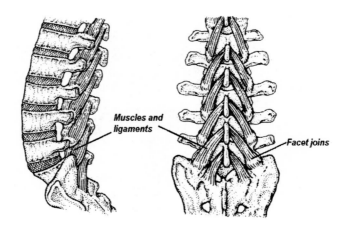

Fig. 9. Inter-vertebral ligaments.

The lowest vertebrae (L5) is supported by a much shorter pair of ligaments and is less flexible compared to the rest. Because this vertebrae supports the rest of the spinal column, it carries maximum weight and thus creates a weak point right at the Sacrum-Lumbar joint, despite additional support from the pelvis internal ligaments.

The longitudinal ligaments

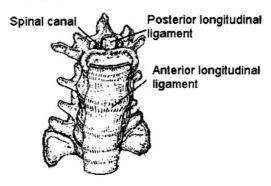

Fig. 10. Longitudinal ligaments.

All twenty-four moving vertebrae are wrapped in two very strong ligaments that run the full length of the spine in the front and the back. These ligaments ensure every vertebra in the spine remains in its proper place. They also limit how far the vertebral column can bend, forwards or backwards. Any distortion or misalignment in the spine creates pressure on these ligaments, causing them to tighten. This can create pressure on any other weak or collapsing disc aggravating its condition. The whole spine can lose flexibility or become rigid.

This condition can be aggravated by muscular spasms triggered when the intelligence in the body detects one or more joints being out of place. The muscle spasms are designed to tighten the muscles around the affected joint in order to protect it from further harm, but the muscle tension may get permanently locked in if not treated properly. The lower the affected joint, the more pressure is created on the ligaments causing the whole spine to become as stiff as ship's mast held rigid by the tight cables. This rigid condition can cause weak discs to collapse.

The nerve connection.
Radiating from the spinal cord is a network of nerves which links the spine to the different parts of the body at different levels. This network originates from the left and right sides of the brain. From there it emerges through the base of the skull and into the spinal column. Individual nerves are formed in pairs and connect to both sides of each vertebral joint or level (Figs. 11& 12). From there they go out to specific organs and tissues in the whole body, right up to the surface of the skin. This network controls the sensory and motor functions of the entire body. Any obstruction or compression of any nerve by misalignment of the vertebrae or any other reason will create pain, lost of sensitivity, and loss of muscle control or functioning in the specific organs or area of the body that the particular nerve is connected to.

As you can see in the following diagrams, the vertebrae are organized into groups: C1 to C7 connect to the Cervical (neck) area, T1 to T12 connect to Thoracic (upper back) area, L1 to L5 connect to the Lumbar region (lower back), and S1 to S5 connect to Sacrum area (bottom of the spine).

The graphics in Figs. 11& 12 may be used to understand the connection between areas of pain or pins and needles and the spinal level from where the nerve branches out of the vertebral column. For example, problems related to specific areas of the foot or leg may be linked to obstruction to specific nerves in the lumbar region. In many cases narrowing of the particular joint may be related to the condition.

These diagrams may help you understand how problems in any area of the spine can cause trouble in different parts of the body. Injury or excessive demand on any vertebrae can produce muscle spasms, which in turn aggravate nerves and create the scenario for problems beyond the area of the spine. Minor problems may be resolved using the *MYOBack* exercises to reset the pelvis and the *MYOBack Roller* exercises to work on individual joints (see Chapter 4). You should always consult a medical professional in the case of serious problems or complications. It is recommended to be well informed and advised before attempting self administered exercises and techniques. Please bear in mind that a nerve that has been giving pain signals for too long may still do even if the cause of pain is removed. Some nerve damages may be irreversible. Then again the older you are the more difficult it becomes to correct or reverse conditions that have been established for too long. For that reason it is recommended to promptly seek advice in any case of long standing pain.

A case of loss of muscle strength.

Rafael Herreros from Chile had been loosing strength on the two smaller fingers of both hands since he was about 20. He was in its forties when he came to see me. The muscles corresponding to those two small fingers were almost non existing. The corresponding nerves come from the base of the neck where the thoracic spine joints the cervical (C8). Rafael had gone through innumerable medical tests and doctors found that his case was quite intriguing as the nerve signal was there however he was still gradually loosing more and more strength as the muscles related continue to disappear. It was obvious that even when the electrical impulses were registered in the tests, the signals to tell those muscles to maintain themselves was missing or too weak. At his age there was little hope to regenerate those muscles but he wanted to stop the deterioration.

Trying to find out the origin of the problem we found that he had a bike accident at the age of twelve. As the front wheel jammed he remembered being catapulted forwards and landing on the ground with his head and neck being pushed up on impact.

On the first session of MYOBack Rafael felt a big jolt at the base of the neck. His posture improved and although there was no miracle cure, the deterioration didn't continue.

As in other cases, Rafael gained stability and went back to live a life as normal as it was possible.

The following full page diagrams represent the nerve connections as looking at the front as well as the back of the body.

Motor and Sensory map (front view)

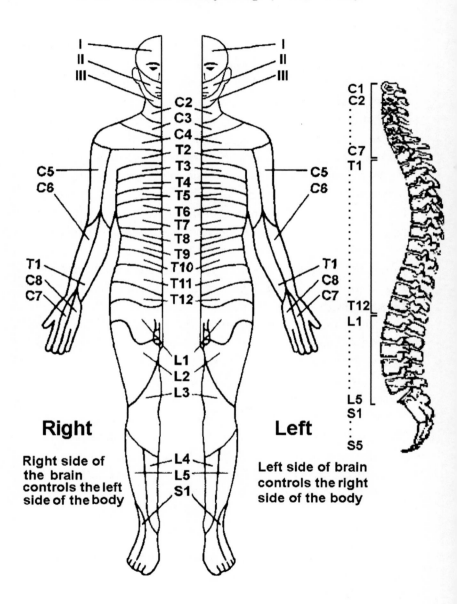

Fig. 11. Motor and Sensory map (front view)

Motor and Sensory map (back view)

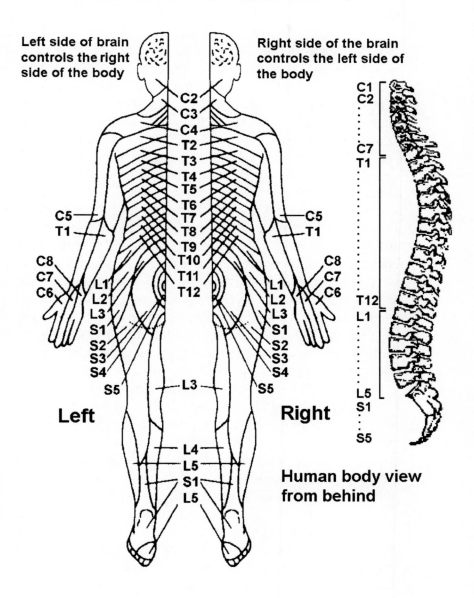

Fig. 12. Motor and Sensory map (back view).

How Modern Lifestyle Causes Back Problems

In today's world, back pain may well be one of the most common health complaints. Modern life style, with lack of proper exercise and too much sitting in unnatural and damaging postures, contributes to all kinds of painful conditions. Long hours of being seated in chair and at desks compresses the spine and causes the shortening of key ligaments and other damage to the pelvis and lower back. As the pressure inside the disc is higher when sitting, the sacral table pushes up under the descending column and the lower vertebrae are trapped in a vertical vice. As the lumbar vertebrae get pushed closer together fluid is forced out of the discs. Most of the fluid is lost in the first hour of sitting but the longer the discs are squeezed the worse they become. Not being able to absorb nutrients and release toxins on a regular basis, the discs will begin to deteriorate and eventually some layers may separate causing hernia. Over time, the combination of too little exercise and too long sitting will cause the discs to lose density. Getting up from sitting becomes a difficult task, as the lumbar region becomes increasingly rigid and fragile.

In addition, the powerful hip flexor muscles at the front of the pelvis will cramp up when compressed for long periods. This causes tightness across the front of the hips and down the legs, which makes it difficult to stand up straight. This affects the positioning of the pelvis which in turn compresses the sacrum-lumbar joints. The pelvis gets tilted backward which throws the whole spine out of balance. The problem is usually compounded by an uneven reaction of the left and right ligaments creating a twist in the spinal column. As the anterior and posterior longitudinal ligaments hold the whole stack of vertebrae in place, stiffness and changes will be propagated throughout the full length of the spine. Tight pelvis flexors can keep your pelvis and lower joints out of place and cause you to take shorter steps, as the legs can't properly angle themselves at the hips.

The combination of poor positioning of the hips plus some twist caused by lower back problems around the sacrum-lumbar can set up the scenario for serious troubles. In such cases, premature wear and deterioration around the hip joints may eventually require hip replacement surgery.

Bad pelvis posture can make you walk twisting to the left or right in order to compensate for poor hip mobility. This can get worse if scar tissue is formed. Scar tissue is extra tissue created by the body to fill up a damaged area, rather like an internal body cast. If allowed to grow too much, it can lock the body into an unnatural position and compound the problem.

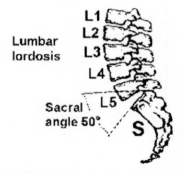

Fig. 13. Alignment of the lower spine

Long hours of arching forwards such as in sitting at a desk, will cause the anterior longitudinal ligament that runs down the front of the vertebrae to tighten like a bowstring and make standing up straight more difficult.

Acting as a vise against the first disc or sacral joint, the pelvis will compress the L5/S1 joint setting the pelvis at a new closer angle with the corresponding ligaments, changing their length and making the new angle more or

37

less permanent. The deterioration will get worse with the passage of time and lack of exercise. The internal ligaments between the pelvis and L5 and L4 will change length aggravating the situation even further and causing more twists and distortions along the length of the spine.

A case of loss of lumbar curve.
Ryan Sharkey, a 30 year-old young Australian man was suffering from what is called "bottom out syndrome" where the lumbar curve is just not there. Ryan was born with severe problems in four vertebrae in the middle and lower areas of the thoracic section of his spine. When he was ten years old, he had to have surgery to fuse these malformed vertebras as they were beginning to fuse together by themselves. Twenty years later Ryan developed a visible lump around the upper area of the fused section of spine, where his poor posture was putting undue pressure. After using the MYOBack technique for a short time, Ryan's posture improved dramatically; he felt taller and more flexible. In just over a month the lump in his spine began to diminish and he could resume normal activity.

Correct Posture

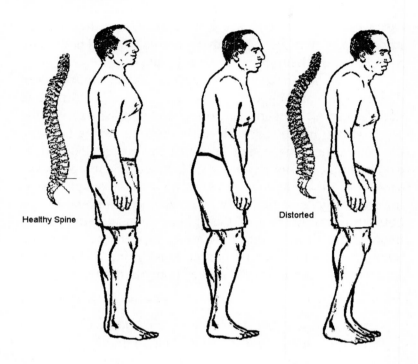

Healthy Spine

Distorted

Good posture   Leaning back   Hunch back

Fig. 14. Changes in the lower joints affect the whole spine.

The loss of the correct curve in the lumbar region is the most common cause of bad posture. The loss of the lower lumbar curve affects the whole spine, as it must keep the balance against the forces of gravity. Degeneration of the joints follows.

Good posture should never be forced. When the body assumes any posture it is because it is trying to accommodate some pain or discomfort. But if the problem is serious then there will be no way to avoid the pain, as the spine carries so many nerves and any interference creates pressure on those nerves. Bad posture can definitely aggravate a condition and can be very damaging, but it is essential to correct the problem before the posture can be improved. Once the problem is corrected, the body will naturally seek the right posture all by itself.

As we age we tend to accommodate injuries and distortions that happen as we go along. Accumulated damage can arise in any part of the spine, most likely at the weakest link in the chain. Because the spine is the home of the central nervous system it is like the power distribution center for the whole physiology. Stiffness or damage in any section of the spine may result in poor nerve supply to the different organs of the body and affect general health. The optimum performance of the spine is considered vital for maintaining good health. If working properly the vertebral column will allow for the proper functioning of the whole spine and will optimize the nerve supply to the whole body.

Helen Gunter was a 75 year-old German lady I met in Switzerland with severe degeneration of the lower spine. When I first saw Helen, I thought her chronic condition was too advanced for the MYOBack technique to be effective, so I told her I was afraid I couldn't be of any help.

Helen, however, insisted she wanted to learn the technique despite all my warnings. She had no doubts that she would come out triumphant. In the face of her resolute spirit, I had no choice but to help her and we agreed to try the technique very gently and with extreme caution, carefully listening to any alarm signals from her body. To my amazement, after only a couple of weeks of practice, she was walking with a feline grace, her chin up and shoulders back as if she were a queen. With a big smile in her face she informed me: "I don't have pain any more."

Scoliosis

Scoliosis is the name given to a condition where a section of the spine is bent or twisted out of its normal balance shape (Fig. 15).

Degeneration in some part of the spine, a shorter leg, or a birth malformation can cause this. As the body must compensate for gravity and create balance in order to maintain posture, it will generate some turn in the opposite way somewhere further up in the spine.

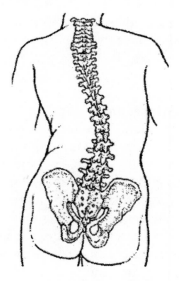

Fig. 15. Typical scoliosis.

Scoliosis is a condition that will require medical advice before attempting to use *MYOBack* techniques. There are many forms and degrees of the condition, some minor some severe. Most health practitioners agree a proactive approach is needed to reduce or minimize the pace of deterioration that occurs with the passage of time.

A case of scoliosis could result in a pair or a number of twists and turns creating weak joints and sections of vertebrae with little movement.

41

After some time the problem can be aggravated by muscle spasms and can cause increasing pain or even lead to a herniated or collapsed disc. In a scoliotic section the joint at the lowest part of it is at most risk as it has to bear the whole weight of the spine at an unnatural angle. A scoliotic section of spine will lose flexibility and become rigid because the cycles of compression and decompression, nutrition intake and elimination of toxins, stops working. Then the deterioration of the joints may lead to severe problems of the whole scoliotic section. In some cases a person can have two or more scoliotic twists in different directions and the disk at the base can be badly compressed.

How best to handle scoliosis

Unfortunately there is no easy way to improve a scoliotic condition without having to go through some pain barriers. Scoliosis pain is mostly generated by muscle spasms and facet joints in the affected areas and you will need to work through that pain to improve the condition. The condition must first be diagnosed by a medical professional who can assess the extent of the condition and what the limitations for exercise and treatment are.

A chiropractor or sports physical therapist can manipulate the vertebrae to restore movement in the affected areas but this does not provide a long-term solution and you end up becoming a slave to a program of regular adjustments.

In the great majority of cases, most experts agree that keeping the affected joints flexible is the best. Plenty of movement and exercises are vital; ignoring the condition will only encourage rapid deterioration over time. It is vital that the affected section of spine gets proper movement to keep the discs healthy through the absorption of nutrients and elimination of toxins. Movement means life, while the lack of it will speed up deterioration and decay.

Most people suffering scoliosis find relief from the *MYOBack* technique and the use of the *MYOBack Roller* or tennis ball rollers (see Chapter 4) If the condition is not too advanced, with patience and regular practice, you may be able to improve the scoliosis section of your back and live with less or no pain. Like most healthy people, people suffering scoliosis do better if they keep a regular exercise program.

Movement and activity are essential
The human vertebral column is meant to be a flexible rod that bends and twists in all directions. Compressing and decompressing the joints allows fluid exchange in each of the joints, eliminating toxins and taking in the nutrients that will keep the joints young and supple like a cat. For this reason, the yogis of India have for centuries practiced yoga *asanas* (postures) and other techniques to make sure the whole of the vertebral column is kept flexible and in tip-top condition. They know that proper alignment and function of the spine is vital for the flow of energy essential for good health and proper evolution in life.

PART II
TAKING ACTION
THE *MYOBACK* TECHNIQUE

Chapter 2
The *MYOBack* technique

Fixing the foundation

Just as a properly laid foundation creates a strong building, correcting the foundation of the spine is fundamental to fixing all back problems. The *MYOBack* technique is designed to create a healthy spine from the bottom up. It begins by resetting the angle and position of the pelvis. Restoring balance at the foundation of the spine naturally corrects the distortions and deviations that aging, muscle weakness and other causes may have created throughout the vertebral column. Resetting the foundation naturally corrects posture and leads to improved fluid exchange in the joints, thus creating spontaneous realignment and more flexibility in the whole vertebral column.

It is not uncommon for problems in the neck, in the buttocks or anywhere in the spinal column to go away after the foundation of the spine is corrected. Many people feel taller, enjoy improved posture and walk more easily after one or two sessions with the basic *MYOBack* exercises.

The *MYOBack* Technique

The initial *MYOBack* exercises are designed to balance the pelvic joint and set it at the correct angle. Once that is achieved, the whole stack of vertebrae is able to spontaneously rearrange itself, resulting in correct alignment and the proper curvature in the *lumbar curve.* If the whole spine can keep its balance against the forces of gravity, the *thoracic* and *cervical* curves also will be correctly aligned. This allows the natural circulation of nutritional fluids into the discs and the natural removal of toxins from the discs. Both these processes and proper curvature are necessary for the maintenance of a flexible and healthy spine.

Further *MYOBack* exercises then stretch and strengthen the whole spine so that the pelvis remains set in the right position and the rest of the spine maintains strength and flexibility.

The *MYOBack* setting of the pelvis is a self-administered, gentle and non-manipulative procedure using only your own muscles and a little help from gravity. You don't have to be an expert yogi to achieve this.

Once the pelvis goes back to its right position, the effect can be quite noticeable, especially if it has been out of place for a long time and there have been long-standing back problems. Better posture and a more flexible pelvis is usually the first thing to be felt. You may feel taller and walk more easily as your legs "hang" more loosely from the pelvis. With further practice, as more tension is released from the joints, muscles and ligaments, you may notice increasing strength in the lower back and throughout the spine. Early hip problems and pain from pinched nerves will likely disappear as the spine finds its natural position and resumes normal functioning. *If this does not occur, then it is likely that you have a more serious problem and will need to consult with a medical expert or a trained MYOBack professional.*

NOTE: The advanced *MYOBack* technique for chronic conditions is tailored to individual needs and is only available under proper supervision. Please refer to the website www.MYOBack.com to find the *MYOBack* professional closest to your home. Once your personal version of *MYOBack* technique has been learned, it is yours to use for life and allows you to become self sufficient in maintaining a healthy spine.

1. Resting your back

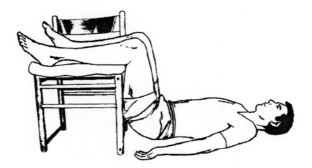

Fig. 16 Resting your back.

Before beginning the exercises to set the pelvic joint correctly, it is good to rest the back completely for ten minutes. In order to do this, lie flat on the floor (you can use a blanket or a thin exercise mat) with your legs resting comfortably on a chair or something similar (see Fig. 16). Use cushions or folded blankets to adjust the correct height so that all weight and tension is removed from the pelvis and your back is as flat on the floor as possible. You can play your favorite relaxing music or chanting (I recommend listening to Vedic chanting).

After resting, the pelvis is engaged by removing the chair away from you while holding your legs up and then stretching them wide apart to about 45 degrees of the floor while pulling with your hands to keep some resisting tension (Fig 17).

It's a good idea though, to keep the chair further away from you so that it's kept between your lower legs/ankles. This will act as a reminder to keep your legs apart during the next step.

2. Engaging the Pelvis.

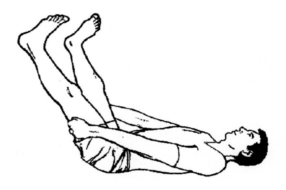

Fig. 17 Engaging the Pelvis

By holding your legs apart and at 45 degrees of the floor you force the leg muscles to keep a good grip on the pelvis. You should feel your leg muscles tight and keep them that way for the next step and until you get them to the floor where you rest them for a couple of breaths before you repeat this step.

To return to the position in step 2 always lift up the knees first by dragging your feet's on the floor and then straighten the open legs at 45 degrees of the floor.

3. Lowering the legs while keeping tight muscles.

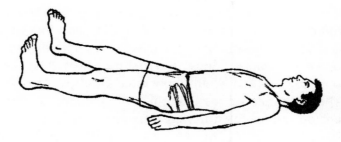

Fig. 18 Setting the pelvis

Then let go with your hands and keep the legs straight and apart and outstretched with tight muscles while you allow them to come down to the floor in about 3 seconds (Fig 19). Allow the legs to lower themselves to the ground at the count of 3 then let them feel heavy and relaxed (Fig 19). Don't lower your legs too slowly, use the 3 seconds count, no longer.

4a. Setting the pelvis 2

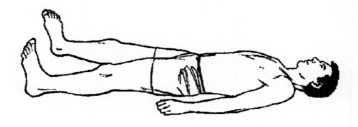

Fig. 19 Setting the pelvis.

The action of gravity and the tension in the leg muscles will lower the pelvis in an even and balanced way. As your legs come down to the ground you may feel tension in a number of muscles or ligaments telling you that they need to stretch or re-arrange themselves. It is not unusual to feel (and even hear) a "clunk" the first time the pelvis goes back to its correct (and healthy) position. Don't worry about this. After a couple of sessions this will probably disappear. If tension is felt down the legs or anywhere around the hips during the setting of the pelvis, it is an indication that certain ligaments needed stretching. This is all very natural and should go away soon or after a few days of the practice. Repeat this exercise five times at the beginning and three times once you feel the improvement.

Warning
Do not lift the legs straight as it will put too much pressure on your low joints.

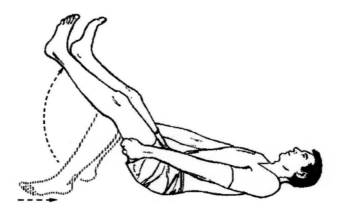

Fig. 20. Caution on lifting the legs.

To return to the legs up position as in step 2 always lift up the knees first by dragging your feet's on the floor and then straighten the open legs at 45 degrees of the floor.

4b. Breathing exercise - Aligning the vertebrae.

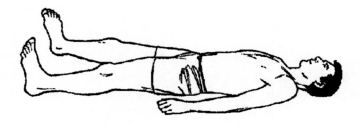

Fig. 21. Breathing exercise.

Once you have completed setting the pelvis three times, remain lying on your back with the legs comfortably apart and straight and take a deep yogic or diaphragmatic breath, gradually expanding the abdomen first and then the lungs, letting the back naturally arch upwards as you inhale. Once the chest is fully expanded, slowly exhale. As the exhalation is completed, try to get your belly down as if you want it to touch inside the spine and push your lower back downwards and try to make your back as flat against the floor as is comfortably possible. Take your attention away from any painful area and just concentrate on making your back as flat as you can. Repeat this yogic breathing exercise five times while lying on the floor with legs apart and flat to the ground. After the pelvis changes position and the sacrum lumbar joint opens up, this exercise enables the vertebrae to naturally fall back into their correct alignment in the spinal column in a domino effect. Take a rest in between as your body needs.

5. Rolling side to side

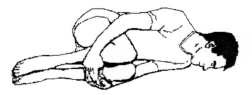

Fig. 22. Sideways rolling exercise.

From the lying flat on your back position, bring both your knees up to your chest and hold them as close to your chest as you can while keeping your head touching the floor. Slowly roll from side to side keeping your hands firmly together over the knees. You should lead with your head and allow the body to follow. Keep the neck relaxed and the head touching the floor at all times. Breathe out as you turn down and breathe in when coming up.

Roll from side to side a five times and return to the starting position, slowly release the arms, and extend your legs out from the hips.

6. Sideways stretch

Fig. 23. Stretching after setting the pelvis

After completing the setting of the pelvis, breathing and rolling exercises, the next exercise is a twisting motion to gain sideways stretch and encourage further re-alignment. Remain lying on your back with your arms and legs apart. I call this the "Star Position". Bring the right knee upward until the foot is level with the knee of the left leg. Keeping the right arm stretched out against the floor, turn your head towards the extended hand. Then slowly lower the right leg down and to the left over the left leg keeping the right foot anchored against the left knee. Stretch as far as it is comfortable. Use your left hand to gently help push on the right knee towards the floor. Only stretch until you feel an easy tension. Don't force the leg further than is comfortable. Listen to the signals from your body telling you how far you can stretch. Hold this position for five full breaths while your attention is in the stretching area. Then slowly return the right leg back to the open legs position. Repeat the exercise, stretching the left knee down over the right leg. Do three sets of this exercise with each leg. If you have been having any pain or problems down one particular leg or one side of the hip, then stretch towards that side first.

This stretching and twisting exercise helps complete the rearrangement of the pelvis/sacrum and loosen up the muscles and ligaments in the pelvic area.

7-8. Activating the pelvic muscles
Sit on your heels with legs close together and toes turned inwards. Have your big right toe over left for men and opposite for ladies. Raise the body slowly upwards as you breathe in while keeping the trunk straight or leaning back slightly to ensure engaging the inner pelvis ligaments. When you are kneeling straight up, rest for a few seconds and then on the out breath slowly lower the body back down until just touching the buttocks to the heels before rising again.

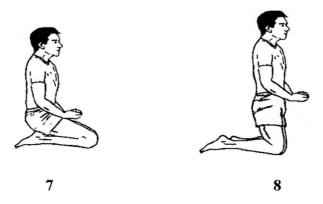

7   8

Fig. 24. Asanas after setting the pelvis

Do three sets up and down, moving slowly all the time as this increases the workload on the pelvic muscles. This exercise is very strengthening for the muscles and ligaments in the pelvic region.

9. Chandra or child asana
From the sitting kneeling position (24.8) raise the arms above the head and slowly bend forward, pivoting from the waist until the hands touch the floor (or as close as you can comfortably get). Keep the legs together and the buttocks resting on the heels so that the pressure is on the stomach rather than the hands. Hold the position for five breaths breathing deeply in and out, feeling the expansion in the lower back as you inhale. Yogic breathing or allowing the stomach to push out will achieve best results.

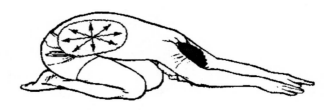

Fig. 25. Chandra or child asana

56

This exercise generates abdominal pressure, which will help to expand the joints and decompress the discs as well as stretching the rear longitudinal ligament. It is vital for the regeneration of those sections of spine that have been compressed and losing fluids for some time. Allow your awareness to go to the stretching of your spine as you fill up the lungs. Notice the stretching going down to the tail bone as you do a little push while the lungs are full. This exercise can also be done with a Swiss exercise ball by kneeling in front of it and then leaning over the top of the ball.

10. Knees to chest.

Lying on your back and keeping your head on the floor, bring your right knee up to your chest and hold it with both hands. Try to place your knee on the center of your chest.

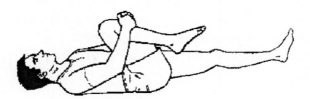

Fig. 26. Knees to chest exercise 1.

Continue to breathe deeply using yogic breathing while you become aware of the expansion that occurs in your spine as you fill up your lungs with air. Hold the position for five full breaths then try to touch your nose to your knee. Hold this position for another two breaths and then slowly let the knee go and allow the leg to go flat on the floor. Repeat with the other knee.

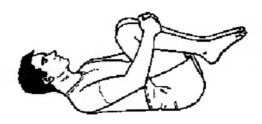

Fig. 27. Knees to chest 2.

Having done both legs separately, pull both knees up to your chest and hold them there. Continue to breathe deep and slow while you become aware of the expansion in the vertebrae that occurs as you breathe in. After five breaths, try to get your nose as close to your knees as possible and hold for two more breaths. Slowly let go of your legs and let them lie flat on the floor.

11. The Cobra (Fig. 28)
Warning. *Due to problems with the facet joints, some people's backs can lock up when bending backwards in the Cobra or similar positions. Avoid these postures if this is the case. Always listen to your body and consult a doctor if in doubt.*

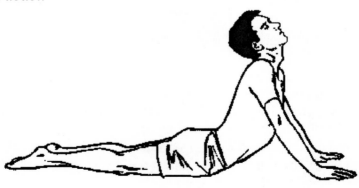

Fig. 28. The Cobra.

This position stretches the front longitudinal ligament. This allows more space between the vertebrae and also tones the muscles at the front of the abdomen.

Lie face down on the floor with the hands flat under or next to the shoulders. Start by raising your head back and up, then slowly push gently with your arms to raise the chest, trying to keep the hips on the floor and lean the head back as far as you comfortably can.

While holding the position, open the mouth fully and stretch the tongue out as far as you can. This is called the Dragon pose. Maintain this pose for five breaths while breathing through your mouth and then slowly let the body down flat on the floor. Rest for a few seconds and then repeat the Cobra and the Dragon. Do this three times.

This completes the *MYOBack* exercises to set the pelvis to its natural position.

12. Rest and body awareness

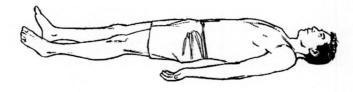

Fig. 29. Resting pose.

You should now lie on you back for two or three minutes and let the mind and body totally relax. Listening to relaxing music or Vedic chanting will be beneficial.

This sequence of exercises can be done every day until flexibility and balance is achieved. Once the pressure caused by misalignments is taken away from the joints and they start to move properly again, the nutrition and elimination cycles are restored in the vertebrae joints. You may notice all kinds of minor sensations anywhere from the very low part of your spine up to the neck as everything starts to get back into balance, but these will soon pass. Over time, with regular practice even totally collapsed discs could be repaired through this method.

Quick setting of the pelvis

Once you have achieved the opening of the low lumbar angle and proper setting of the pelvis you can do a quick setting of the pelvis as you feel the need to do so. Engage the pelvis by lying on your back with your legs apart and lifting up the legs by bending the knees up first. Straighten the legs up in the air while keeping them wide apart. Hold the legs in that position for a few seconds to encourage the leg- pelvis joints to firmly engage and then lower both legs slowly and evenly until they touch the floor. Then you do a quick twist to each side, holding for three breaths.

Some people may have a tendency to get loose quickly and should be careful not to over-stretch. If that is the case, once the pelvis is reset and loose the full resetting sequence should not be done every day. *MYOBack* should not be overused as it is a very powerful technique. In that case it is recommended to do only a quick setting of the pelvis followed by a good set of asanas or sun salutations at least once a day once flexibility and buoyancy is achieved.

You can then do the full *MYOBack* program when you feel you need it.

Remember that healing takes time. Due to the poor blood supply and fluid exchange, the misaligned or damaged joints may take some time to be repaired or restored. It may take up to nine weeks for a real and permanent change to take place. During this time you might experience some "setbacks". Be patient and continue the program!   Eventually the new structural changes will become permanently integrated into your physiology.

The following full page diagrams are designed as a worksheet to help your MYOBack technique practice.

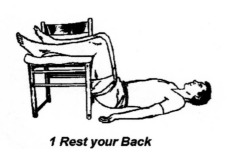

1 Rest your Back

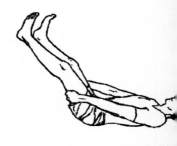

2 Engage the Pelvi

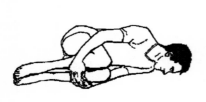

5 Rolling Side to Side

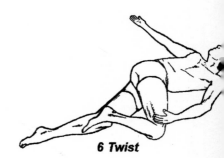

6 Twist

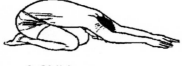

9 Child pose

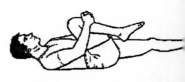

10 Knee to Chest

Worksheet 1 – The *MYOBack* technique

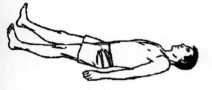

3 Set the Pelvis 1

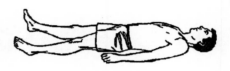

4 a Set the Pelvis 2
4 b Breathing

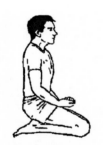

7 Sit on Heels

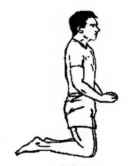

8 Rise

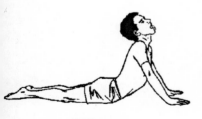

11 Dragon

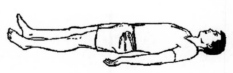

12 Rest

Chapter 3
Strengthening the Back

Once you have corrected the position of your pelvis and opened up your lower joints and propagated the realignment up the spine, you need to develop the key muscles to make these changes permanent. The first *MYOBack* exercise (Fig. 30) reinforces the pelvic muscles and ligaments, as well as developing strong abdominal muscles. This is essential in order to maintain the proper abdominal pressure required to keep the discs in the proper cycle of compression and decompression. The second exercise (Fig. 31) strengthens both the neck muscles and the inner pelvis ligaments. Both exercises use the law of gravity, to ensure proper pressure, balance and control.

Caution. *These exercises are designed to be used only after the resetting of the pelvis has been achieved. Some are very demanding, require a minimum level of fitness and should be approached carefully, building strength gradually over time. Unfit individuals may need to go to a gym or consult a personal trainer first. If you have a severe back problem, scoliosis or any complication, it is recommended that you only do a mild version of these exercises and leave a few days between each session, to allow your muscles to rest properly. Abdominal exercises can adversely affect joints that are weakened. Please seek medical advice if this is the case before attempting these exercises.*

Abdominal exercises

There are many well known abdominal exercises and here you can see a couple of simple but effective examples.

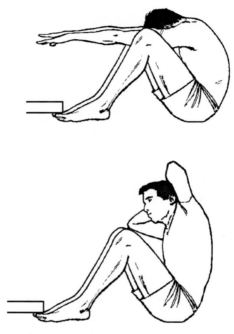

Fig. 30. Abdominal exercises

Lie on your back with your arms in front and your raised knees. Squeeze your abdominal muscles so that your lower back and your upper back, shoulders and head rise in a rowing-like movement. Repeat, doing as many curl ups as comfortable, with a 10 seconds rest every 30.

Then you can try the same with your hands behind your head and elbows out in a curl up, with twisting motion, alternatively touching your right or left knees with your elbows. If you are over 40, any abdominal exercises may cause some compression of the discs. If your muscles are weak, try to build up your strength slowly. Too much too soon can undo the benefits achieved with the setting of the pelvis. On the other hand, you need to exercise, otherwise you will continue to get weaker and more out of condition. You can get some relief from the compressing effect of the muscle building exercises by ending the session with a full or even a quick setting of the pelvis, including the sideway stretching, after setting the pelvis as in Fig 21.

The *MYOBack* upper back exercise.

Just as with the *MYOBack* abdominal exercises, in the upper back exercise you will be developing strength in a whole range of muscles. The idea is to make the strong muscles of the neck stronger. I call this exercise a "backwards push-up." *Again, if you are too weak to do this exercise, then you should be extremely careful and at first only tense the muscles with the intention to do them allowing time for your body to build up strength before attempting the full exercise. Consult a medical practitioner if you have serious neck problems or doubts.*

Make sure that you have the right nutrition for your body to build up muscles. This is very important. You can consult a nutritionist to make sure you have a balance diet.

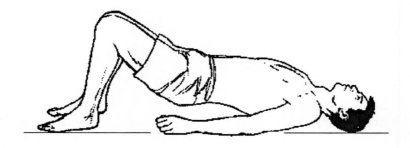

Fig. 31 The *MYOBack* upper back exercise –
"Backward pushups".

Lie on your back with the legs slightly apart and the knees drawn upwards. Use a small cushion under your head, to make it more comfortable. Tense up the muscles with the intention to lift up the body, by using your strong back neck muscles first. Once you have developed the strength you can attempt a brief backward push up. With your arms on the floor, push your whole body up, keeping the neck and back straight, so that your whole weight begins to be supported by the back of the head. Use a cushion or pillow under your head. Don't put undue strain on the neck. To begin with, use your elbows on the floor to support your head. Eventually, when you are strong enough lift your arms from the floor; use them only to keep your balance.

It is not unusual to experience some strange sensations or even discomfort in the neck muscles at the beginning of this practice. Again, you must listen to your body and go one little step at a time. If you have had a previous neck problem, you may notice new muscular sensations that are different from the old pains. The old pains will probably fade away, even if the new pain remains for a little while.

Build up the number of backward pushups until you can do up to ten sets each session.

With both these exercises, you will be able to test how well you are doing, by feeling the muscles and ligaments over the front of the pelvis. They will tighten up and feel stronger.

The *MYOBack* abdominal exercises

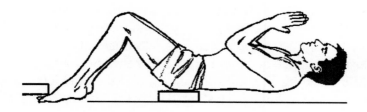

Fig. 32. The *MYOBack* abdominal exercise.

The *MYOBack* abdominal exercises are very demanding and only suitable for fit people. They are recommended as an addition to the above simple abdominals. You activate many muscles in a very short time.

Lie on your back with a thick book under the base of your spine and your toes tucked underneath a sofa or chest of drawers for leverage. Press the palms of your hands together to create pressure across the chest muscles and slowly lift your upper body a few inches from the floor, keeping the spine and neck straight. Holding that position and keeping the hands pressed together, slowly touch the ground with the right elbow, without twisting the upper body. Slowly return to the center position and then slowly move in the opposite direction and touch the left elbow to the ground, while holding the body off the floor and without twisting the torso. Return the hands to the center position and maintaining pressure in the hands gently lower the upper body to the floor. Rest for few seconds. Resting is equally important as exertion for building strength.

Then do the same sequence again, but this time keeping the hands pressed together, slowly touch the ground with the *left* elbow first, without twisting the upper body. Slowly return to the center position and then slowly move in the opposite direction and touch the *right* elbow to the ground, while holding the body off the floor and without twisting the torso. Return the hands to the center position and, maintaining pressure in the hands, gently lower the upper body to the floor. Rest for few seconds.

Repeat the exercise, except this time grip hands tightly together and try to *pull* them apart throughout the exercise. Raise the upper body and hold a few inches from the floor while touching first the right elbow and then the left elbow to the floor, without twisting the torso. Gently lower the body to the floor and rest.

Then do the same sequence again, but this time touching the *left* elbow first and then the *right* elbow to the floor on the next without twisting the torso. Gently lower the body to the floor and rest.

This is one set of the *MYOBack* abdominal exercises. Start by doing one set each session and slowly increase the amount over time, until you can do up to ten sets each session. Don't be surprised if you find them hard to do to at first. I met a young athlete named Shujaa who found the *MYOBack* abdominals difficult, even though he could effortlessly do 130 normal abdominal crunches without a break. If you cannot raise your body off the floor, then it's a sign your muscles are very weak and you will need extra time to develop your strength. Don't rush. Slowly exercise in order to improve your condition. Be cautious and only try the exercises once every few days.

Abdominal exercises, such as muscle building exercises, won't just build stronger muscles but also encourage the body to reduce fat tissues and improve overall health.

How to use traction with the *MYOBack* abdominal exercises.

If the *MYOBack* abdominal exercises seem to undo the benefit of the setting of the pelvis and you are not so young any more, there is a good chance that abdominal exercises are compressing the weak discs in your spine. In that case you can include traction in the practice. You can use a board on an angle, with your head lower than your feet so that your body weight creates traction at the same time that you are doing your ***MYOBack*** abdominal exercises. The lower your upper body and head with respect to your feet, the more traction will be generated by the action of gravity. See Fig. 33

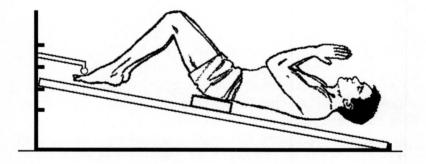

Fig. 33. Abdominal exercise including traction.

Performing the ***MYOBack*** abdominal exercises will not only develop strong abdominal muscles for better support. It will also send a signal to the body to keep strong bones to go with the strong muscles. This in turn will prevent or help reduce Osteoporosis.

71

Leg stretching to prevent back problems

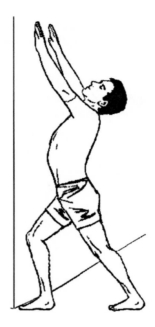

Fig. 34. The Runners Stretch No. 1

Your leg muscles, tendons and ligaments are very powerful and can alter the pelvis position creating problems in your spine. A tendon not exercised properly will tend to get shorter and tighter. Runners know how important it is to keep stretching so that you keep the proper flexibility and the legs hanging freely from the hips. The following stretching exercises can help maintain flexibility and strength in the legs.

In the first exercise, face the wall with the front of both feet touching the wall. Stretch both arms upwards. Keeping the right foot touching the wall, reach the left leg backwards. Keeping the toes of your back foot pointing straight forward, place your full weight on your back foot (Fig. 34). Hold for ten to thirty seconds as you feel the tension at the back of the leg. Repeat the process switching the positions of the legs.

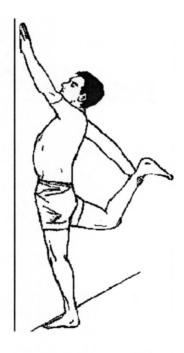

Fig. 35. The Runner's Stretch No. 2.

Still facing the wall, reach upwards with your left arm. Grab your right ankle with your right arm and pull your leg back until you feel the tension at the front of the leg (Fig. 35). Hold this for ten to thirty seconds then repeat with the other leg. You will find that you get looser with practice.

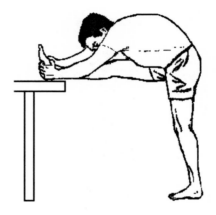

Fig. 36. The Runners Stretch No 3.

Place your right leg on a chair or low table. Reach forward with both hands and grab hold of your ankle (or as close as you can reach (Fig. 36). Hold the position for ten to thirty seconds keeping both legs as straight as possible and feeling the tension. Repeat the exercise, switching legs. You can work your way up to a higher table as you become more flexible.

The following full page diagrams are designed as a worksheet to help your MYOBack strengthening exercises practice.

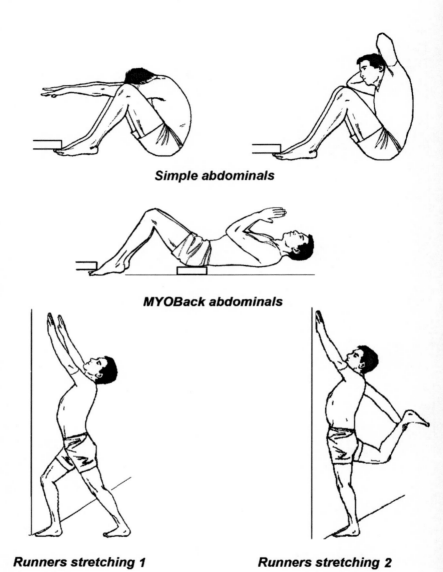

Simple abdominals

MYOBack abdominals

Runners stretching 1　　　　**Runners stretching 2**

Worksheet 2 – Strengthening exercises

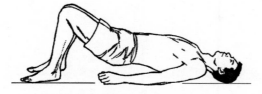

MYOBack backward push ups

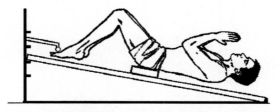

MYOBack abdominals with traction

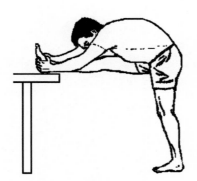

Runners stretching 3

Chapter 4

Exercising and Massaging the Spine Using a *MYOBack Roller* and Gym Balls

A *MYOBack roller,* tennis balls and gym balls can be used effectively to exercise and massage the spinal joints as well as to locate areas where there are muscle spasms, misalignments or other problems. You can improvise a simple roller by using two hard tennis balls bound tightly inside a cotton sock. The most effective roller, however, is the *MYOBack Roller*, which is specially designed for this purpose (Fig. 37). This will be available from the website www.myoback.com.

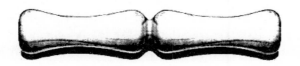

Fig. 37. The *MYOBack Roller.*

NOTE: If you have scoliosis or muscle spasms, try the tennis balls first, as they apply a gentler pressure than the *MYOBack Roller.*

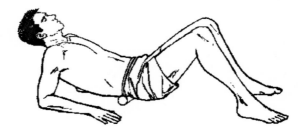

Fig. 38. Using a *MYOBack Roller.*

Lie on your back on the floor with your knees raised. Place the roller under the lower back with the raised parts on either side of the spine. Raise the body up, supporting yourself on your elbows, and slowly move the spine up and down the roller, gradually proceeding up the spine in a backward and forward motion. You can adjust the pressure to a comfortable level by raising or lowering the body using the elbows (Fig. 38).

This will provide a good deep massage to every individual joint and promote fluid exchange in the discs to remove toxins and help keep them healthy. While doing a general massage with the *MYOBack Roller,* too much pressure applied on any one point can be damaging, so maintain continual movement while using the roller and rest whenever you feel the need. If you encounter a tender or painful spot, it means there is a joint that is jammed and could be on its way to collapse. Typically one side will hurt more than the other. When a joint is stiff, there will be tight and sensitive muscles in that area. You can massage those muscles by going up and down over them for up to 30 seconds at a time. Don't be surprised if you develop slight bruising in those areas of your back. Getting a stuck joint to move may take some time and work, but with persistence the joint will loosen and the pain will diminish.

Always listen to the signals coming from your body and adjust the treatment accordingly. If necessary, take a break from using the roller for a couple of days, or if you are using the *MYOBack Roller*, switch to the tennis balls inside a sock for a little time as this will be softer on the painful area. If the painful joint gets worse or it doesn't change over time you may have a damaged facet joint so don't persist.

This rolling is also good for the thoracic area. For that you can go a bit flatter, with the knees higher up in order to move the pressure upwards to massage the upper back. When using the *MYOBack Roller* on the upper back and cervical regions, you can also support the weight of your body by placing your hands over your head and on the floor to support your weight.

Using the roller to treat a collapsing disc

A seriously collapsing disc will cause severe pain when rolling over it and will usually be accompanied by nerve pain such as pins and needles or numbness in the areas supplied by the affected nerve. You may want to start with tennis balls until the pain goes down. The pain will generally be felt on the opposite side of the body to where the nerve damage is. If you locate such a problem, you should roll up and down the affected area slowly. Depending on the severity, you can do this for a few days and then you can stop. Once you locate a tender spot, stop the roller there for a few seconds and allow it to sink into the affected joint. This way you will be opening up the joint and decompressing the disc to allow the nutrients to flow in as well as getting the facet joints to move. If comfortable, you can do this for a little more time each day. If it becomes uncomfortable, take a break for a few days and then continue.

Once you can tolerate holding the roller in that place for a while, slowly try moving your knees to the right and then to the left in order to achieve some lateral movement of the affected joint. Once you have finished using the *MYOBack Roller*, you can slowly do the *MYOBack* spinal twist a couple of times on both sides to get a good stretch. Don't be surprised if you feel some cracking as you do.

Once the muscles that have been in spasm let go, you may feel instability in the joint. In this case, it is good to be gentle and use light pressure while using the roller. Be patient. Given time, massage with the roller will allow the joint to recover its flexibility and buoyancy.

The first time a locked joint move could be dramatic and could trigger some inflammation or even spasm of the joint, or the nerves and muscles around it. It may be wise to stop treating yourself for some time to allow the inflammation to settle down before continuing.

After several sessions the tender, jammed segment will become less sensitive and some pleasant sensation may arise in the area. We call this "good pain" and it is a sign of healing taking place. The real test on how well you are doing with your self-applied therapy is how well you feel during the rest of the day.

How well and how quickly a joint recovers depends upon a person's age and how bad the injury or deterioration is. Healthy, fit people have a better chance of recovery. Lack of exercise and improper nutrition impede recovery because they cause discs to become weaker and softer.

Stretching after using the roller

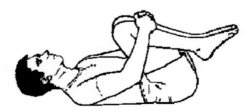

Fig. 39. Knees to chest exercise.

After using the roller, you should do some stretching exercises or yoga asanas (see Chapter 2) to encourage proper alignment and expansion of the joints. Lying on your back on a yoga mat or folded blanket, pull up your knees to the chest and hold for at least 30 seconds while breathing deeply in and out (Fig. 39). This will create abdominal pressure that will help to expand and decompress the discs. Next, rock backwards and forwards on your spine (Fig. 40).

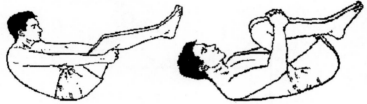

Fig. 40. Rocking backwards and forwards on the spine.

Rocking on your low and high back area on a yoga mat will provide a good massage and encourage movement in the vertebrae. Then you can do the child pose (Fig. 25) and the cobra or dragons pose (Fig. 28).

Using Gym Balls

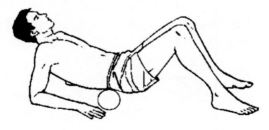

Fig. 41. Back roll using a gym ball.

Once the back feels free of sensitive spots, gym balls can help to maintain movement and flexibility.

A basketball-sized ball that is not too hard can be used to roll the full length of the back, providing a healthy massage that will keep all vertebrae moving (Fig. 41). This is not a substitute for the *MYOBACK Roller*, but it will help.

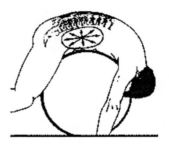

Fig. 42. Using a large gym ball.

A large gym ball (55 to 65 centimeters or larger) can also be used to help the expansion or decompressing of the spine. There are many books or videotapes available showing other useful exercises to do with gym balls.

The need to exercise
Lack of exercise is the surest way to create problems in your back. Lack of movement in the vertebrae and weak muscles will lead to deterioration and stiffness and rigidity in the joints and eventually to collapsed or herniated discs and fused vertebrae. And, of course, a lot of pain.

Once you start with the *MYOBack* technique, it will be good to see a professional personal trainer to get help in assessing and strengthening the weak parts of the physiology. Apart from the *MYOBack* exercises, get yourself on a regular exercise and strengthening program. You will find all the exercises much easier to do once you have corrected the imbalances in the spine with the *MYOBack* technique.

Chapter 5
The Need to Exercise

As you grow older the body starts to receive subtle signals to go into a state of dissolution. Similarly, if you don't exercise, the body's natural intelligence will start reducing muscle cells, replacing them with fat cells or letting the muscles shrink and wither away. Bones also begin to reduce and calcium is eliminated at a higher rate. So we need to constantly remind our bodies that we still need muscle strength and functionality. We do this by regularly exercising and making use of the muscles, tissues and bones.

The internal organs also benefit from proper exercise. You may have experienced how better the digestion is if you take a good relaxing walk after you have eaten.

Every kind of exercise should be practiced with moderation, especially as you get older. Each of us has a different physiology and thus different requirements for exercise. No single exercise routine is suitable for everybody, neither is there one diet to fit all. In the science of Ayurveda, this is taken into account, not only for exercise regimes, but also for diet and lifestyle recommendations. Having a good relationship with your body and its requirements is vital for a long, happy and healthy life. Wise men will tell you the mind and body should be good friends and agree to look after each other. We will talk more about this in Part III of the book.

If you haven't been exercising much recently, it would be advisable to go to a gym and consult a professional trainer for advice on how to get yourself back into regular exercises. You may need to develop certain muscles to regain your overall strength. A gym is a good place for low impact aerobic exercise and also for weight training (preferable under qualified guidance). Those of you, who are getting older, should not try to take up any new sport without consulting a good trainer first, though it is generally okay to resume a sport you grew up with as your body is used to the physical requirements.

Aerobic exercises

Aerobic exercises raise the metabolic rate and accelerate the heart functioning in a controlled manner. The main benefit is opening of the arteries and strengthening the heart muscles. If you want to keep a water pipe running smoothly and free from obstruction, the best way is to flush the pipe out regularly with extra water flow to remove sediment build up. This is similar to the effect that raising the metabolic rate has on the heart.

Running or jogging is not recommended as the hard impact of the feet hitting the ground can send shock waves into the body, which can damage the ankles, knees, the uterus in ladies and even the brain. More gentle aerobic exercises such as swimming, biking, rowing, etc. are better.

Muscle building exercises

Muscle building exercises usually include putting pressure on or tensing muscles using increasing weight loads and many repetitions. This sends a message to the body's intelligence center that more muscle mass is required. Some basic muscle-building exercises are included as part of the *MYOBack* technique (Chapter 3).

These are intended to strengthen those muscles needed for a healthy back. Other exercises will be needed for other parts of the body.

Muscle building exercises also play an important role in maintaining healthy bones, and to fight osteoporosis. In many cases, osteoporosis has been reversed using muscle-building exercises. In 1993, I was having problems with my left hip and was diagnosed with poor bone density. The hip was suffering rapid deterioration and was frequently jamming, and I was in constant pain. I was heading towards hip replacement surgery.

This all happened at the same time as I was having my worst lower back problems. I was told my condition was triggering calcium loss throughout the body and I was offered drugs to force the body to retain calcium. I refused them because I thought it would be like twisting the body's arm to force it to accept something that, for some reason, it wanted to eliminate.

For me, this was a turning point. I was a firm believer in the natural intelligence of the body. If my body wanted to get rid of its calcium, there must be a good reason for this. So I decided to find out more. I tried to build a friendly relationship with my body. The idea was to find peace rather than declaring war. From then on, there would be no more punishing the body but rather looking for ways to make it happy.

Soon after that I cognized and developed the *MYOBack technique.* This allowed me to solve my hip problem by resetting the pelvis in the correct position. Then I started a series of muscle building exercises to give me the strength to maintain the pelvis and the rest of my vertebrae in their right positions. Bliss flooded my body as the old pains and suffering was forgotten. Fourteen years later, at the age of sixty-five, I had to have surgery to repair multiple breaks in my left femur bone following a serious car accident. The operating surgeon was amazed to see how strong my hip bones were and also how quickly I was able to recover from the injury and regain my strength.

The Ayurvedic Approach to Exercise

Ayurveda includes a series of stretching exercises, more commonly known as Yoga, whose aim is not merely to flex the body, but more to create harmony (the term "Yoga" literally means union) between mind and body. From a spiritual perspective, this means infusing intelligence or consciousness into the physiology in order to unite the gross and subtle aspects of human beings. In recent years, yoga has become increasingly popular in the West, as people search for solutions to our stressful and materially oriented way of life.

Yoga postures (called *asanas*) are a series of stretching exercises that help maintain and improve the body's flexibility. At the same time, they open subtle channels in the physiology to allow the proper flow of energy and the elimination of toxins (known in Ayurveda as *ama*). *Ama* includes not only toxic chemicals in the physiology but also impurities in the mind, which lead to dullness and mistakes in the thinking.

Yoga exercises play a key role in maintaining a flexible and healthy spine. They specifically benefit the cycles of compression and decompression of the joints, which as we have discovered is vital for the elimination of toxics and introduction of nutrients. Seated poses help to create stability and optimal spinal alignment after the pelvis is properly seated and good posture. Forward bends stretch the longitudinal ligament, stimulate digestion, increase the spine's flexibility, and calm the physiology. Backward bends create mobility and flexibility in the spine, especially in the upper back, and at the same time are invigorating to the whole body. Inverted poses stimulate the endocrine system and allow for increased circulation, while poses, which twist the body laterally aid digestion, elimination, and tone up the spinal column. The resting pose brings increased awareness, orderliness, and balance to both mind and body.

There are many different forms of Yoga available. Most are generally well tolerated by just about everybody as long as they are practiced gently and without straining the body. You don't have to tie yourself in knots to achieve the benefits. Stretching should only be done to the limits of each person's body. With practice flexibility will gradually increase.

Some of the Yoga exercises presented below are already included in the *MYOBack* exercise program. However, here they form part of a specific routine and can be performed as a set. It is best to practice these Yoga exercises after performing the *MYOBack* exercises.

NOTE: *The Yoga exercises presented here are a basic set for guidance that will help anyone be able to maintain flexibility throughout their body and especially in the spine. When beginning Yoga practice, it is recommended to consult first with a trained Yoga instructor. Due to specific structural problems, pregnancy, overweight, acute illness or menstruation, etc., postures may be adjusted to serve one's particular requirement. Most cities now have plenty of trained Yoga instructors available.*

Basic Yoga Exercises (15-20 minutes, moving slowly)

A few points to remember before practicing:
>   **a)**   Ayurveda recognizes that energy flows differently in male and female bodies. For this reason, men should always start exercises and massage on the **right** side of the body, while females should begin on the **left** side.
>   **b)**   To be practiced morning and evening (ideally before sunset).

c) Wear comfortable, loose clothing. Use a non-slip flat surface that is not hard. You can use a folded blanket, rug, exercise mat, or any other semi-soft surface. Choose a quiet place where you will not be interrupted. Disconnect the telephone, switch of the cell phone and don't have the TV or radio on, or even soft music in the background. Just let the mind be easily aware of the body in silence.

d) It is important to follow the prescribed sequence of postures because it is designed to warm up the body and remove stiffness. Then it gradually progresses towards invigorating, strengthening, and stretching the entire body. Also, each pose is a preparation for the next one or a counterbalance to the previous one.

e) Perform the postures slowly and without pushing the body beyond its comfort zone. Hold each posture for about 30 seconds and then release slowly and easily. Never move in or out of a posture suddenly. Use the breath to facilitate the movement.

f) Be gentle. There is no "ideal" pose, as everyone's body is different. If you can't touch your toes without undue effort, it doesn't matter. If necessary, bend the knees slightly to ease stretching until your flexibility improves. In each posture, take the body to the point where you can begin to feel the stretch and no more.

g) Allow your awareness to naturally go to the area of the body that is being stretched (very important). The mind as well as the body is involved in all Yoga exercise. Use of the attention facilitates the removal of accumulated stress.

h) Be patient, it is not a race. Progress comes with practice. Over time you'll notice the increased strength, flexibility, and liveliness that come from the integration of breath, movement, and awareness.

i) Breathe naturally and easily while practicing the exercises. Breathing should follow the body's needs. Inhale and exhale without holding or controlling the breath in any way. When the posture compresses the stomach it is natural to want to breathe out and when your body arches back, it naturally wants to breathe in. Just go with the flow. Breathing should be easy, fluid, and continuous.

NOTE ON BREATHING: *Breathing is something we have all done since birth. However many of us acquire bad habits that are not in accord with what Yoga would consider natural breathing. Breathing in should begin low in the abdomen and move upwards. If you want to see natural breathing, watch a small baby. First the abdomen appears as if it is filled with air, then the chest. Pushing the stomach out will make the diaphragm (flat muscle) to go down. This makes good sense since the lungs are triangular in shape, so it is best to begin with the larger area at the base and then fill the lungs with air from there upwards.*

1. AWARENESS POSE (Chetasana) (At least 1 minute)
It is always best to start with a minute of relaxation. Lie down on your back with the legs slightly apart and your arms spread out a little away from your body with the palms of your hands facing up, so that your whole spine rest evenly on the floor. Close your eyes and allow your body to become heavy and relaxed. Let yourself completely relax as you disengage yourself from your daily activities. Rest for at least one minute breathing free and easily.

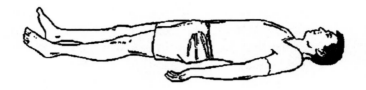

Fig. 43. Awareness pose (Chetasana)

Benefits: This pose is invigorating and refreshing for both the body and the mind, removing fatigue and soothing the entire system. You can return to this pose any time you feel like it during the performance of Yoga asanas or in between each pose.

2. TONING UP EXERCISE (2 minutes)
Toning the body

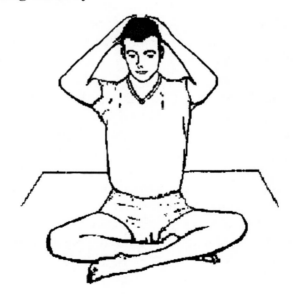

Fig. 44. Toning up 1.

Sit in a comfortable position on the mat. Using the palms and fingers of both hands, press down on the top of your head and then release, repeating the pressing and releasing motion as you move your hands down the front of your head, face and neck and towards the heart. Repeat the procedure down the back of the head and neck to the front of the chest and finishing at the heart.

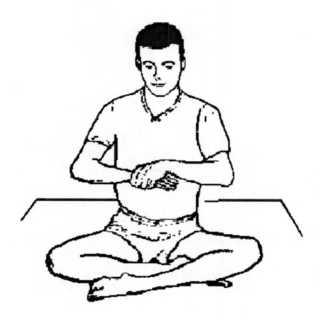

Fig. 45. Toning up 2.

With the left hand begin the squeezing motion on the fingertips of the right hand and gradually move up the arm and across the chest to the heart. Ladies should begin with the right hand on the left arm. Repeat the process on the other arm (left for men, right for ladies). The pressure should be firm and the press and release motion gradual and continuous. Make sure to massage both the top and underside of the arm.

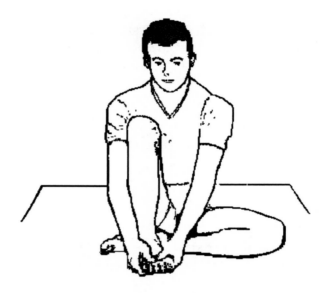

Fig. 46. Toning up 3.

Repeat the procedure on each leg, beginning with the right leg for men and the left leg for ladies. Bring your palms up to your navel and with both hands on the belly; begin to press and release around the abdomen, gradually moving up to the heart. Putting your hands around your back, repeat the squeezing motion around the lower back, kidneys and ribs, moving the hands around the front and up the heart.

Benefits: Toning up directly stimulates the nerve endings under the surface of the skin nerves, increases blood circulation, and is beneficial for the lymph system, which helps eliminate toxins from the body.

3. SIDEWAYS ROLLING EXERCISE

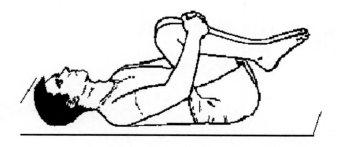

Fig. 47. Sideways rolling exercise 1.

Lying flat on your back, bring both the knees up to your chest and hold them as close to your chest as you can while keeping your head touching the floor. Slowly roll from side to side keeping your hands firmly together over the knees. You should lead with your head and allow the body to follow. Keep the neck relaxed and the head touching the floor at all times.

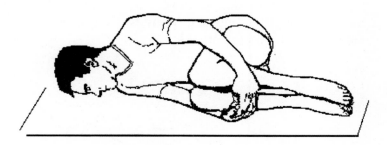

Fig. 48. Sideways rolling exercise 2.

Roll from side to side five times. Return to the starting position, slowly release the arms, and extend your legs out from the hips. Lie flat on your back in the Chetasana and let the body be completely relaxed for a few seconds.

Benefits: Stretches and stimulates the muscles and ligaments in the whole back.

4. KNEES TO CHEST EXERCISE.

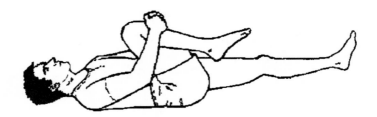

Fig. 49. Knees to chest exercise 1.

Lying on your back and keeping your head on the floor, bring your right knee (left knee for ladies) up to your chest and hold it with both hands. Continue to breathe normally while you become aware of the expansion that occurs in your spine as you fill up your lungs with air. Hold the position for 30 seconds then try to touch your nose to your knee. Hold this position for 10 seconds and then slowly let the knee go and allow the leg to go flat on the floor. Repeat with the other knee.

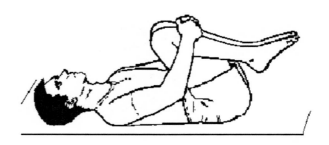

Fig. 50. Knees to chest 2.

Having done both legs separately, pull both knees up to your chest and hold them there. Continue to breathe normal while you become aware of the expansion in the vertebrae that occurs as you breathe in. After 30 seconds, try to get your nose as close to your knees as possible and hold for 10 seconds. Slowly let go of your legs and let them lie flat on the floor in the Chetasana.

Benefits: Encourages the decompression of the discs and absorption of nutrients.

5. SITTING UP POSE (Vajrasana)

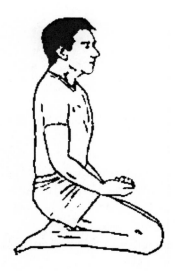

Fig. 51. Sitting on your heels.

Begin by kneeling down with your buttocks on the heels with the back straight up and the hands resting gentle one on top of the other on the lap palms facing upward (right hand on top of the left for men and left over right for ladies) (Fig. 51). The feet should be slightly apart and the right big toe crossed over the top of the left toe (Left toe over right toe for ladies).

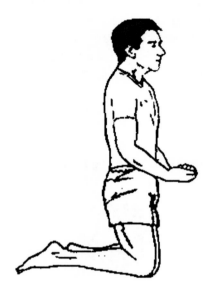

Fig. 52. Coming up to kneeling position.

The head and neck should be straight up as if they were held from the ceiling by an invisible string. Look straight ahead and breathe normally. As you inhale, slowly lift your buttocks off the heels with the torso straight up or leaning back slightly. Keep the spine extended and the chest out with relaxed shoulders (Fig. 52). Hold for a few seconds. Exhale and slowly lower the body without leaning forward and sit back on your heels. Move slowly throughout, keeping your body nice and relaxed and breathing deeply and easily. Feel the pelvis muscles working hard. Repeat five times.

Benefits: Strengthens the pelvic region, removes tension from the knees and ankles, and helps to build up a strong foundation for the lower back.

6. CHILD POSE (Chandrasana)

After finishing five repetitions of the Vajrasana, remain sitting on the heels with the knees together and raise the arms above the head with outstretched fingers as far as you can. The hands should be touching slightly.

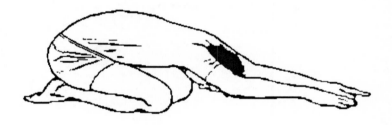

Fig. 53. Child pose.

Keeping the arms outstretched, lean forward, pivoting from the hips until the hands touch the floor (Fig. 53). The weight should be supported by the stomach on the knees rather than the hands on the floor. Breathe deeply in and out while holding the pose for at least 30 seconds. Feel the spine expanding from the pressure in the abdominal cavity as you breathe in.

Benefits: Expands the vertebrae and allows nutrients to flow into the discs.

7. HEAD TO KNEE POSE (Janushirsasana)

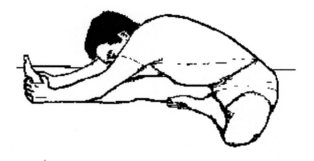

Fig. 54. Head to knee pose.

Sit down with your legs slightly apart and extending out in front of you. Point your toes upwards so you can feel the stretch in the back of the legs. Bend the right leg and place the sole of your left foot against the inside of the right thigh (Ladies bend the right knee and place the sole of the right foot against the inside of the left thigh). Keep the outside of the knee flat on the floor (Fig. 54). As you inhale, lift up your arms over your head and straight up in the air with the hands slightly touching. Exhale slowly and bend your body forward, hinging yourself from the hip. Keeping the arms straight out, reach forward and try to touch your right toes (left for ladies).

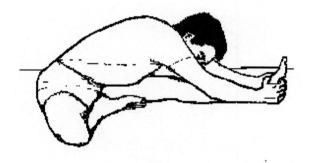

Fig. 55. Head to left knee.

Keep your upper body as straight as you can and your lower back relaxed. Don't strain. Go only as far as you comfortably can. Hold the pose for a few breaths, then, as you inhale bring your arms back up above your head, keeping them straight the whole time. Stretch towards the sky and breathe in as deeply as you can. Reverse legs and repeat the exercise (right leg bent for men, left leg bent for ladies), moving slowly and steadily the whole time (Fig. 55)

Benefits: Strengthens and relaxes the spine, stretches the sides of the discs, tones the abdomen, liver, and spleen, and aids in digestion and elimination.

8. HALF SHOULDER STAND (Sarvangasana)

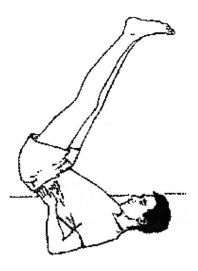

Fig. 56 Half shoulder stand.

Warning: *Perform this posture slowly. If you have a chronic back problem or high blood pressure, be sure to check with your doctor before attempting.*

Lie on your back and press your arms and hands flat against the floor. Let the shoulders relax and stretch out your spine. As you exhale, bend the knees and slowly raise the legs over your head. Use your hands and elbows to form a stable platform supporting your body (Fig. 56). Stretch your legs over your head, keeping the torso bent to avoid too much pressure on the head and neck. Breathe normally and let the body relax. Start by holding the posture for 30 seconds and gradually increase to 2 minutes if you are comfortable in the pose.

Benefits: Promotes movement of encephalic and other fluids, plus the entire endocrine system; has a soothing effect on the body, bringing flexibility to the spine, relieving mental fatigue and increasing circulation to the thyroid gland.

9. PLOW POSE (Halasana)

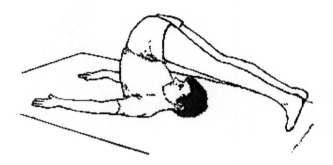

Fig. 57. Plow asana.

From the Sarvangasana you can flow directly into the Halasana posture. As you exhale, bend from the pelvis bringing both legs down over the head and allowing your legs to go as far down towards the floor as you comfortably can without straining and where you can still breathe. Make sure not to put too much strain on your neck. If you feel any pain, slowly raise the legs and come out of this pose.

Once you have comfortably achieved the Halasana, you can fold your arms over your head and hold the pose for a few breaths. Hold the posture for 15 seconds at first, increasing to one minute as you get more comfortable in the pose.

Come out of the posture as you exhale, using your hands to support your lower back. With the knees bent, slowly lower the legs to the floor. Take a few moments resting in Chetasana.

Benefits: Strengthens and relaxes the neck, back, and shoulders and promotes movement of encephalic and other fluids.

10. COBRA POSE (Bhujangasana)

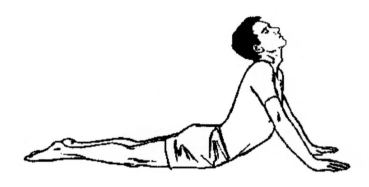

Fig. 58. Cobra.

Warning: *You may have problems doing this asana if your pelvis is not properly set up or have degeneration of the lumbar region. Never force the body and avoid this posture if you sense your back locking up.*

Lie face down with your forehead touching the floor. Bring your feet together and place your hands on either side of the face with the fingers pointing forward. Keeping your head steady and looking forward, slowly roll your head upwards, then your neck and chest in a continuous movement. As the chest rises, take a deep breath, press firmly down with the hands and expand the chest outwards, keeping your elbows close to the body the whole time. Stretch your head and neck well above your shoulders and away from your ears. Imagine your head being pulled up towards the ceiling by an imaginary string. Hold the breath for a few seconds and then exhale as you slowly lower your body back to the floor. Relax for a few seconds lying face down before repeating the movement. Repeat this pose some three times.

Benefits: Stretches the front longitudinal ligament of the spine, promoting expansion of the discs and more flexibility. It is also helpful with uterine and ovarian problems.

11. LOCUST POSE (Shalabhasana)

Continue lying face down. Stretch your arms down by your sides, either under the thighs or next to your hips with your palms facing upwards. Bring both feet together and rest your head on your chin. Feel the whole spine stretching. As you exhale, raise one leg upwards and back as far as you comfortably can while keeping the leg stretched out. Hold for a few breaths and then slowly lower the leg back down. Then do the other leg. Be careful not to hold the breath while doing this pose. Repeat the pose some three times. If it is easy, you can then once raise both legs at the same time and relax. Men start with the right leg, women with the left.

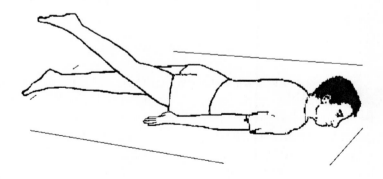

Fig. 59. Locust.

Benefits: Strengthens the lower back muscles, aids digestion, and benefits the bladder, prostate, uterus, and ovaries.

12. THE TWIST POSE (Marichyasana)

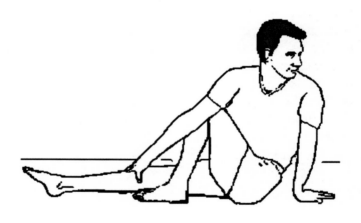

Fig. 60. The Twist.

Sit with the legs extended straight out in front of the body. Keep the spine straight, the head tall and neck loose. Bend your left leg keeping the sole of your foot on the ground. (Ladies start with bending the right knee). Bring your heel just above the inner part of your right knee and toward your buttocks. The inner side of your left foot should be touching the inner side of your outstretched right thigh. Putting your arm outside your left knee, grasp your right knee with your right hand and hold firmly. Inhale, stretching your spine straight upwards. As you exhale, extend your left arm out in front of you and twist your body to the left, pivoting from the base of your spine. Keeping your eyes fixed on your left hand; allow your head to follow your arm until you have twisted as far to the left as you can. If it is comfortable, bring your left hand around your back and onto your right thigh. Go only as far as you can without straining. Keep the spine straight throughout this posture and avoid bending forward.

Breathing normally, hold the posture for a few breaths. Release slowly and then repeat the exercise on the other side. It is very important to use your breath in this posture and only twist during exhalation.

Benefits: Stretches the disc walls and helps to realign all the vertebrae; it also increases circulation to the abdominal organs, relieves tightness in the upper back and shoulders, stretches the neck, and stimulates the liver, kidneys and adrenal glands.

13. BENDING FROM STANDING POSITION (Uttanasana)

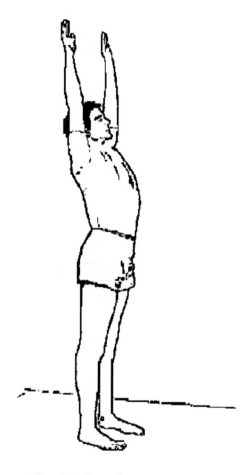

Fig. 61. Standing up pose.

Standing up as straight as you can with your feet a few inches apart and pointing forward, lift you arms straight up in the air and stretch towards the sky as far as you can (Fig. 61) as you inhale deeply. Let your chest open up and your head and neck straight up and relaxed.

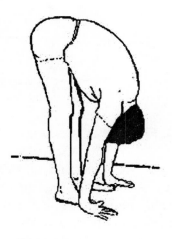

Fig. 62. Bending down pose

On the exhalation, bend the body forward from the waist. Allow your knees to be loose and bring your hands to the floor (Fig. 62). Keep your shoulders and elbows relaxed and don't lock the knees. Hold the pose for a few seconds as you breathe easily. As you inhale, lift up your arms up, again pivoting from the waist. Come all the way up until your arms are stretched up over your head. Exhale and lower your arms down to the sides.

Benefits: Tones the entire spine, the liver, stomach, spleen and kidneys; soothes and cools the mind.

14. AWARENESS POSE (Chetasana)

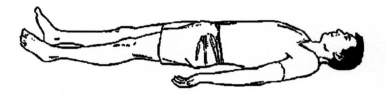

Fig. 63. Resting (Chetasana).

Lie down on your back so that the whole spine rests evenly on the floor. Allow your legs to relax and stretch away from the pelvis, and let the feet drop open to each side. Arms should rest loosely next to the body with palms facing upward. Close your eyes and let your body completely relax, allowing any tension to release from the neck, shoulders and hips (Fig. 63). Breathe easily and freely. Maintain this position for at least 60 seconds.

Benefits: Invigorates and refreshes both the body and the mind, removes fatigue, and is soothing for the entire system.

The following full page diagrams are designed as a worksheet to help your Yoga exercises practice.

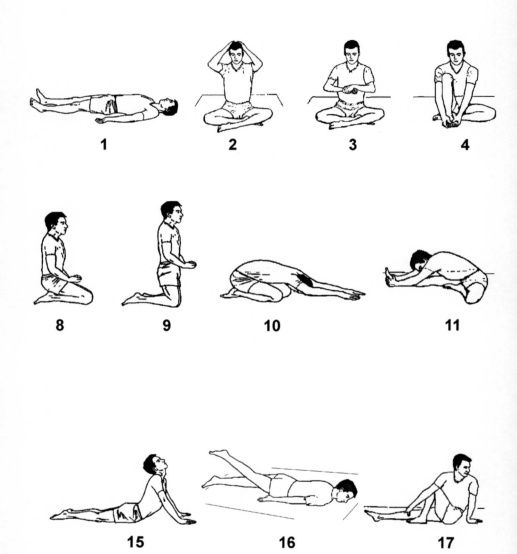

Worksheet 3 – Yoga asanas

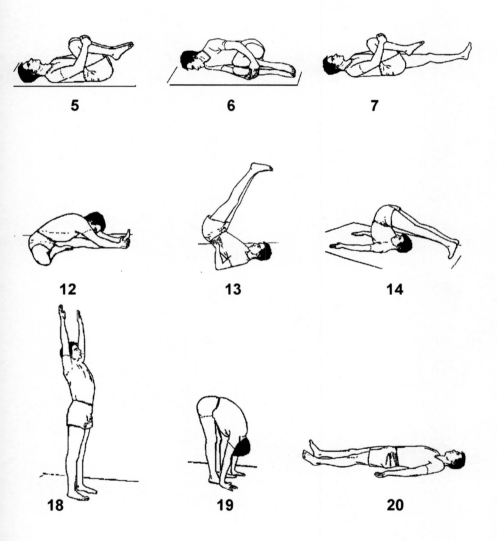

5 6 7

12 13 14

18 19 20

SUN SALUTATIONS (Suryanamascara).

Ayurveda also recommends a special set of exercises called *Sun Salutations* (*Suryanamascara*) designed to invigorate and energize, and create a strong and flexible physiology. This set of exercises is recommended once you have resolved any major problems in your body and shouldn't be practiced if you still have a chronic back condition. If in doubt, consult your physician or trainer.

Suryanamscara exercises are thousands of years old. As the name indicates they are always performed facing in the direction of the Sun, which gives energy to all living things. Face East from midnight until noon, and West from noon until midnight. These exercises are practiced in a continuous flowing fashion, moving from one posture right into the other, and connected by the inward and outward breath. The movement follows the breath and the breathing should flow smoothly and easily. Breathe out when the abdomen is contracted or you are bending forward, and breathe in when the chest is expanded or the body stretched out.

The following pages show the Sun salutation step by step.

1. Salutation (Samasthiti).

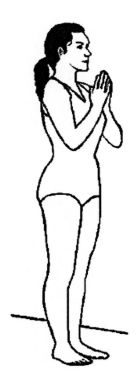

Fig. 64. Salutation

Stand evenly with the feet together and raise the head upwards so the whole spine feels stretched. Place the palms of your hands together in front of your chest. Look straight ahead and expand the ribcage on the inhalation. Close your eyes and allow the breath to be free and easy. Wait for the body to settle down and let you know when it is ready to begin.

2. Raised arm position (Tadasana).

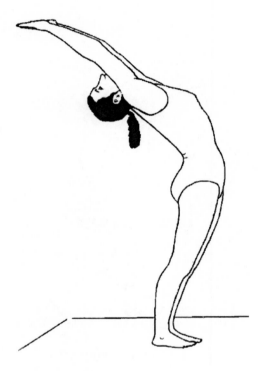

Fig. 65. Raised arm position.

Open your eyes inhale and slowly extend the arms over the head. Lift and expand your chest as you stretch the spine. With your head backward, look straight upward.

3. Hand to foot position (Uttanasana).

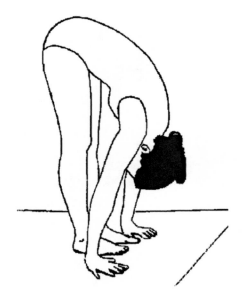

Fig. 66. Hand to foot position.

As you exhale, bend the body forward and down from the hips, stretching your spine, arms, and neck. Letting the knees bend freely without locking, bring the hands to the floor, or the best you can do without straining. Hands should be shoulder width apart and touching the floor outside of the feet. Avoid collapsing your chest or over rounding your upper back. Keep the elbows and shoulders relaxed.

4. Equestrian position (Ashwa Sanchalanasana).

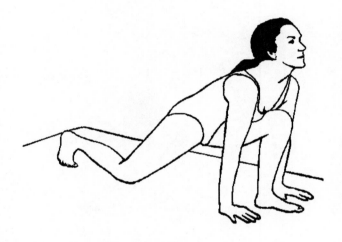

Fig. 67. Equestrian position

As you inhale, extend the right leg back (left leg for men), and drop the back knee to the ground. The front knee is bent and the supporting foot remains flat on the floor. Simultaneously lift the head and spine backwards and open up your chest. Allow the head and neck to elongate vertically.

5. Mountain position (Adhomukha Svanasana).

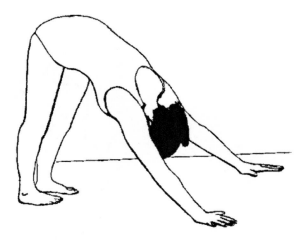

Fig. 68. Mountain position.

As you exhale, bring the front leg back to meet the other leg, with both legs at hip width apart. Hands remain at shoulder distance. As you raise the buttocks and hips, press down with the hands, allowing the spine to release upward and back. Stretch the heels down with your feet flat toward the floor and feel the stretch through the backs of the legs as the body forms an inverted V. Keep the head and neck free and relaxed.

6. Eight limbs position (Ashtanga Namaskara).

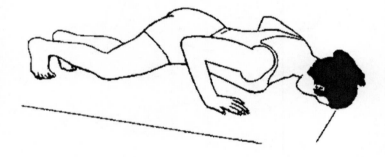

Fig. 69. Eight limbs position.

While holding your breath gently drop both knees to the ground and slowly slide the body down so the chest and forehead also touch the ground. You will have eight parts of the body touching the floor: the toes, knees, the chest, the hands and the forehead. Hold this position only briefly and then continue to move into the next pose.

7. Cobra position. (Bhujangasana).

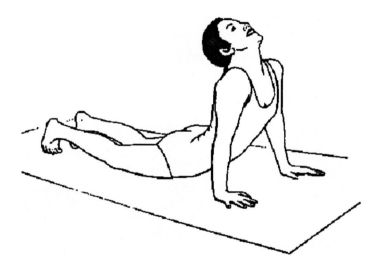

Fig. 70. Cobra position.

As you exhale, roll the head upwards and expand the chest forward and upwards as you press down with the hands. Keep the elbows close to the body and extend the head and spine upward. Open the chest in a continuous movement and keep the shoulders down and away from the ears. Try to look at the ceiling for maximum stretching.

8. Mountain position (Adhomukha Svanasana).

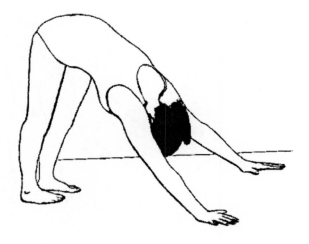

Fig. 71. Mountain position.

Continuing the flowing movement, as you exhale, move back into the Mountain position (Fig. 71) with the body forming an inverted V shape. Raise the buttocks and hips, press down with the hands, and allow the spine to release upwards and back. Keep the feet flat on the floor and feel the stretch through the backs of the legs. Keep the head and neck free and relaxed.

9. Equestrian position (Ashwa Sanchalanasana).

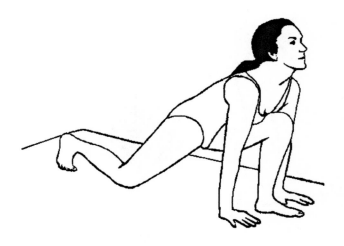

Fig. 72. Equestrian position.

As you inhale, swing the left leg forward between the hands (right leg for men) back into the Equestrian position (Fig.72) but reversing the legs. The right leg stays extended back, knee to the ground (left for men). The front knee should be bent with the foot flat on the floor. Extend the spine, lifting the chest forward and up. Allow the head and neck to extend upward.

10. Hand to foot position (Uttanasana).

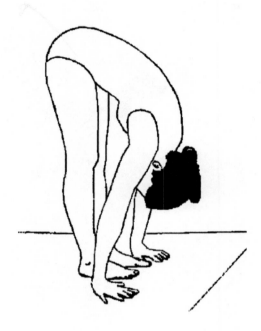

Fig. 73. Hand to foot position

As you inhale exhale, step forward with the right leg and into the Hand to Foot position (Fig. 73). Both hands should remain on the floor. Let the knees soften or bend freely. Avoid collapsing the chest or over rounding the upper back. Keep the elbows and shoulders relaxed.

11. Raised arm position (Tadasana).

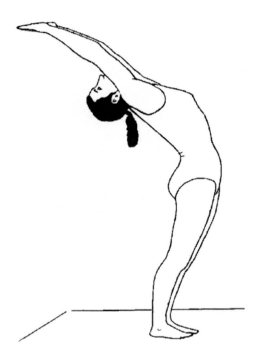

Fig. 74. Raised arm position.

On the inhalation, lift up the arms up and bend the body backwards, pivoting from the hips, and into the Raised Arm position (Fig. 74). Continue to lift and expand the chest as you come up, extending the arms back over the head.

12. Salutation position (Samasthiti).

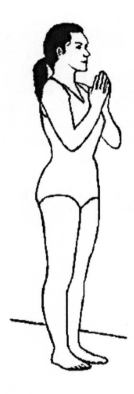

Fig. 75. Salutation.

Exhale as you lower the arms and bring the palms of your hands together in front of your chest in the Salutation position. Stand tall with the feet set naturally apart at hip width. Fill the chest with air and expand the ribs as you look straight ahead as you stretch the neck and head upwards. Hold the Salutation position while breathing naturally for a few breaths while you wait for the body to settle down.

From the Salutation position move directly into the second cycle using the alternative leg stretched back in the Equestrian position. This completes one cycle of the Sun Salutations.

You can do as many repetitions of the Sun Salutations as comfortable up to twelve full cycles. You should never go past the point of where the body becomes over-heated from the exercise.

Apart from what we have covered so far you should also look at all areas of your life, including your diet, work habits and lifestyle etc. In the next section of the book we will take a look at some of the things you can do to create balance in every area of your life.

The Ancient Yogis of India understood the importance of maintaining a flexible and healthy spine not only for ongoing health and vitality but also for spiritual growth and evolution.

The following full page diagrams are designed as a worksheet to help your Sun salutation practice.

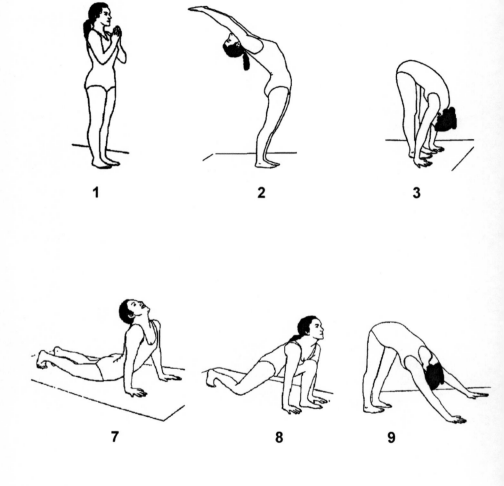

Worksheet 4 – Sun salute

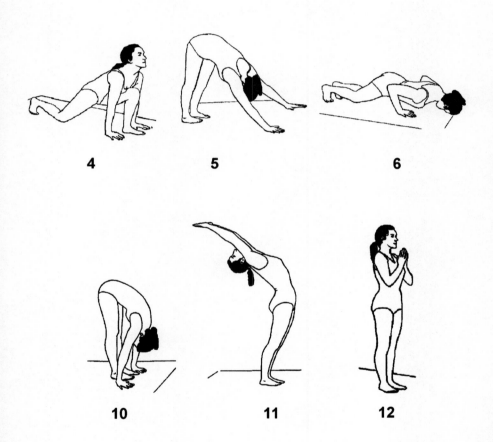

4   5   6

10   11   12

PART III

LIVING WITHOUT PAIN:
A VEDIC APPROACH TO LIFE

Chapter 6
The Miracle of Ayurveda

My mother's remarkable recovery

In 1995, I received news from Chile that my mother's health was declining. At the time I was attending part time classes at Maharishi Vedic College (MVC) in Melbourne. I decided to go home and see if there was anything I could do to help. I had been impressed with what I had learned in my studies at MVC about the holistic approach to health of Ayurveda and I was keen to see if it could help my mother. As I was about to leave, Steve Griffith, founder of Australian Aid for Cambodia Foundation (AACF), a non-profit organization funding educational programs in Cambodia, asked me if I could break my journey to pay a short visit to their university near Phnom Penh. I had been helping acquire inexpensive computers to donate to the University, which had been founded to help some of Cambodia's poorest orphan children get an education. The first shipment of computers was due to arrive shortly and Steve wanted me to oversee their arrival and train the people how to use them. "Are you sure?" I said. It meant going around the world in the opposite direction to get to Chile, a much longer journey. "Yes," he insisted. I didn't know the divine hand of Mother Nature was at play.

When I arrived in Cambodia, it turned out the two people assigned to work with me on the computers were both experts in Ayurveda! They were able to give me an enormous amount of knowledge about this ancient system of natural medicine, which proved to be an enormous boon for my mother. By the time I reached Chile I knew I had been blessed with the knowledge I needed to help my mother. I felt like I had the powers of a magician.

When I arrived, I met with Dr. Silva, the man in charge of treating my mother and a well-known endocrinologist. He informed me that my mother was suffering multiple complications, mainly resulting from old age, that had caused intestinal paralysis and she had no more than a few weeks left to live. Her condition was extremely fragile and there was nothing left he could do. I asked for his consent to try an Ayurvedic approach, explaining that it was a holistic system of medicine thousands of years old that used multiple approaches, including natural herbal medicines, to re-enliven the natural intelligence of the body so the body can heal itself. Given that he had run out of options, he graciously gave me his consent.

I explained to Dr. Silva that the first step would be to facilitate the elimination of toxins from my mother's body. This would allow the natural intelligence of the body to flow properly. I was amazed at the number of pharmaceutical concoctions my mother was taking. How can the body be expected to heal with so many poisonous chemicals being pumped into it? Dr. Silva agreed to suspend almost all drugs my mother was taking, keeping just one for the heart.

To my delight (and Dr. Silva's mystification), my mother showed signs of improvement from day one; at the end of the first week she had gone through a total transformation. The swelling went away, her color returned, and elimination became better than normal. At the end of four weeks, she was not only healthy, but also looking thirty years younger. So dramatic was the transformation, her friends had difficulty recognizing her when they saw her walking around town again. They had been preparing themselves for her funeral and now she was walking around looking better than ever!

As part of her "miraculous" recovery, my mother learned the Transcendental Meditation technique, which plays a key role in Maharishi Ayurveda in connecting the mind and body with the inner source of intelligence, and is extremely effective at removing stress and strain from the whole system. She took her meditation very seriously and practiced it every day for the rest of her life.

My mother enjoyed another ten good years. When she finally passed away, she radiated a blissful peacefulness that affected everyone around her. The priest at the funeral service commented how envious he was to see such heavenly serenity. These days, when there is so much fear of death, is hard to believe a departure could be such a smooth and happy experience, but this is the way it should be for everyone when they leave this world.

Timeless Vedic wisdom and the quantum human body

Thousands of years before modern medicine discovered the mind-body connection, the Vedic sages had developed an "inner technology" that operates from the most profound levels of our awareness. This inner technology connects the mind and body to the source of divine intelligence deep within human consciousness. It is this quantum level of intelligence that creates everything in the universe. By connecting with this source of intelligence through deep meditation, we enliven nature's intelligence in every area of our lives. This, I believe, was the principal reason for my mother's amazing recovery.

According to Ayurveda, understanding and being in tune with this quantum level of functioning is the key to a balanced and healthy life and is far more powerful than any drug, diet, or exercise.

Living in tune with nature

The goal of Ayurveda is perfect health, including freedom from chronic back pain. Perfect health (and a pain free back) depends upon perfect balance in all areas of your life. Everything you eat, say, think, do, see, feel and perceive through your five senses affects your overall state of balance. It would seem impossible to control all of these different things at once, but just as all parts of as tree emerge from the one root, by contacting the quantum source of human intelligence deep within the mind, it is possible to manage everything effortlessly from one place. Perfect health can be defined as living in tune with all the laws of nature. The quantum field of intelligence deep within our own minds is also the source of the laws of nature that govern the whole universe, so from there it is easy to be in tune with Natural Law. To achieve this, the deep silence of meditation where the mind and body transcend day-to-day activity and settle down to their most fundamental level of functioning, is required. This is why it is such an important part of the Ayurvedic approach to balanced health.

Accumulation of toxins and back pain

Another significant factor in maintaining health according to Ayurveda is the proper elimination of toxins from the body. As already mentioned, the general term for toxins in Ayurveda is *Ama*. *Ama* can be either physical or mental in nature. Every influence that enters the body either through the senses as sound, vision, taste, smell or touch, through emotional experiences, or through the consumption of food creates a biochemical response that has to be processed and digested thoroughly by the body. For example, when you have to brake suddenly in your car to avoid hitting someone, the body produces a rush of adrenalin in order to heighten your ability to respond in a timely fashion and avoid danger. Those chemicals have to literally be absorbed and "digested" by the physiology. Any toxic remains have to be eliminated so the mind and body can return to normal functioning. If not, then toxic residues accumulate, restricting the natural flow of intelligence and ultimately poisoning the entire system. The human physiology is remarkably resilient, but if toxins are allowed to build up, over time the system begins to break down and serious illnesses will result. Back pain, joint pain and arthritis-type diseases are typical of the health problems caused by deficient digestion which results in poor elimination of toxins.

Emotional stress

Many back pains are a physical manifestation of emotional worries and psychological stresses that remain deep within our subconscious mind. How do we take on these stresses?

Let's say a five-year old boy makes a drawing that he believes is the ultimate work of art. He shows it to his seven-year old brother only to receive a devastating put-down: "You can't draw", says his brother, showing him a much better drawing he has just done. The little boy goes away and tries again to impress his brother. "You're stupid, you can't even draw," says the great art critic. Taking a different approach, the little boy tries to impress his mother with his beautiful drawing, only to find she is furious with him for doing it on the living room wall and he ends up being punished again. Time passes by and the boy is now twenty years of age. He gets an invitation to an art exhibition, but he refuses, saying, "I am not really interested in art".

There may be no recollection in the young man's mind about how this particular dislike was originally planted in his mind. Only the feeling remains that he doesn't like art. Fear of spiders, dogs, claustrophobia, and any kind of phobias are generated in the same way. There is generally no recollection or thought related to it – just a feeling. These mental traumas or stresses sit in a deep level of our conscious mind and interfere with our ability to act in a natural manner. They materialize as physical impurities in the cells in the body and they can be as damaging to us as any chemical toxins that may ultimately affect your health.

Many of the New Age psychologists, doctors and thinkers recommend positive affirmations to counter-balance the accumulated mental negativity. While this may sound alright on the surface, it would be the equivalent to trying to balance your little boat which is tilting one way due to its load of negative rocks on one side by loading it with positive rocks on the other side.

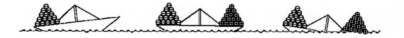

Fig. 76 Overloading your boat.

The end result is you may sink your boat or at least it becomes so heavy that it is hard to sail it through turbulent waters.

Of course it is better to think positively rather than negatively. But to intentionally overload your subconscious mind at a superficial level in an attempt to wallpaper over deep emotional stresses just won't work. A manipulated positive mood that has no real base will crumble at the first challenge and the personality may suffer damage as a result.

Today, people are taking tranquilizers, drugs, pain-killers, smoking cigarettes, drinking alcohol, watching TV, hugging teddy-bears, etc., in order to feel less emotional pain. They want to cover up the problem rather than find ways to remove the mental toxins responsible for them feeling so bad. It requires mental and physical purification.

The Three Gunas

God's creation is a coexistence of interacting forces. Vedic wisdom identifies three primary elements or impulses at work in this universe of complementary energies—*sattva, tamas,* and *rajas*—which directly relate to our mental and physical make-up as well as to our environment and so are vital to our understanding of how to maintain a balanced state of health. These three elements emerge from the state of the Absolute or Infinite, the primeval and unbounded state of creation, which is unmanifested.

Sattva (mostly closely translated as purity) governs the impulse to evolve and move forward in life. *Tamas* (inertia or dullness) is the exact opposite and governs the impulse to stay the same or even go backwards. Emerging from the interaction of these two opposites is *Rajas* (movement), which governs the interplay of *sattva* and *tamas* and is the primary impulse for action. In order for balance to be maintained in the universe, these three forces need to be in a state of equilibrium. We can think of *sattva* and *tamas* as the positive and negative poles in electricity. When they interact a current of electricity (*rajas*) flows between them.

These three impulses, *sattva, tamas* and *rajas*, are called *gunas*. In Ayurveda, they are also used to describe the principal mental body types and are responsible for creating different tendencies in people's lives. Those with *sattva* dominant, for example, like to evolve. Their minds focus on directions that are creative, life-supporting and healthy and they do not care for action for its own sake alone. People with more *rajas* influence in their mental make-up, on the other hand, like to be involved in action and are very much goal-oriented. Their minds are constantly busy and they tend to be restless, impatient and impulsive. Those whose minds have a predominance of *tamas* tend to procrastination, inertia, lethargy, negativity and materialism. They like things to stay the same and they enjoy set routines.

Ayurveda also describes three elements (called *doshas*) relating to our physical body and our environment. These are *vata* (movement, cold, dry), *pitta* (metabolism, hot, dry), and *kapha* (structure, cold, unctuous). Each of us is made up of a different combination of these three subtle elements and so has individual requirements for our diet and lifestyle. Good health is a matter of maintaining proper balance of the *gunas* and *doshas* within the context of our own personal constitution. God made all of us distinctly individual, and although the force of evolution in life naturally takes all of us towards a state of purity or *sattva*, it is important that we go along with nature's unique plan for us. With the overall goal of moving towards a state of optimum health and happiness, it is important that each of us eat, act, and behave according to our own individual nature. In Vedic Science this is known as *Dharma* (right action). Following *Dharma* is regarded as the most successful thing one can do in life to achieve contentment.

Self Health Care

Although Ayurveda has regimes for dealing with all kinds of chronic health conditions, its main focus is on prevention. According to Ayurvedic doctors, the greatest contribution to health is achieved by following proper daily routines of rest and exercise, diet and lifestyle. In other words, self-health care is valued far more than doctor-oriented health care. For self-health care to be effective it has to account for your particular mental and body type and your individual health needs. The best way to formulate your own health care program is to first consult a properly trained Ayurvedic practitioner. They can help identify your *guna* and *dosha* make-up and give you specific recommendations for diet, lifestyle and related herbal formulas. It is a natural step-by-step process that helps restore balance and create health. It should be easy for you to understand and follow and much of it can be self-administered at home.

Here are some general guidelines that will benefit everyone, whatever their individual constitution:

Exercise moderately and regularly

The key to exercise is regularity. You don't have to do a strenuous workout five times a week to stay fit. You can exercise efficiently without straining your muscles. Walking is excellent physical exercise for everyone and beneficial therapy for the heart and mind as well. It is better if you can walk near rivers, lakes or the ocean, as the air will have some additional vitality and freshness (referred to as prana in Vedic Science). An early morning walk for about thirty minutes is ideal. It will not only help your heart, it will prepare you for the day by charging up your metabolism and improving your circulation.

Eat right

Arguably the most critical step you can take towards good health is to eat a good diet. For a society addicted to fast food and eating-on-the-go, this is probably the most difficult habit to maintain. Eat fresh, healthy food (if possible grown organically). Avoid processed foods or genetically modified (GMO) foods. How you eat is as important for health, longevity and heart as well as what you eat. Eat moderately. According to Ayurveda, the ideal amount of food at a meal can fit in two cupped hands. Don't skip meals and, if possible, eat at the same time each day. This helps train your digestion system to anticipate food and thus digest it properly.

Don't overload your digestion by eating a heavy meal at suppertime or by eating late at night. Favor eating before the sun goes down. That way the body is able to process the nutrients and eliminate toxins at night while you sleep rather than having to digest excess food.

Vitamin and mineral supplements may be necessary for optimum health. Research has shown that many of the natural food components we enjoyed when we "lived off the land" are now missing in our diets. We are suffering from a nutritional gap caused by the modern processing of our food supply. We enjoy the ease and convenience of mass food distribution, but the trade-off is eating foods that are devoid of their natural energies, overheated, hydrogenated and artificially preserved. Two of the most serious dietary deficiencies cited in current scientific literature include essential fats and fiber. So called "good fats", essential fatty acids are necessary for intercellular health. Without these essential fatty acids (they are called "essential" because the body cannot manufacture them), our bodies are also unable to properly absorb fat-soluble vitamins such as A, D and E.

It is also important to have abundant dietary fiber, *lignans*, (*see Footnote*) and naturally occurring *probiotics* (friendly bacteria) to promote a healthy digestive system. You can also help digestion with fresh ginger, salt and lime. Taking *lassi* (a blend of fresh yogurt and water) after your lunch is also very beneficial. Blend three parts cool water with one part fresh yogurt. You can add fruit juice or spice it with roasted ground cumin and fresh cilantro for flavor.

[Footnote: Lignans are naturally occurring chemicals widespread throughout the plant and animal kingdoms. Typically, these naturally occurring chemicals cannot be reproduced accurately in the laboratory, even though pharmaceutical companies may claim they can be.]

Recently, *Newsweek* magazine called Omega-3 "the best of all possible fats" and cited flax seed as an important source. The essential oils in flax seeds will oxidize rapidly after being exposed to the air, so the best way to take it is to grind them fresh each day (two or three tablespoons of seeds in a coffee grinder is plenty).

Essential fatty acids (Omega-3 and Omega-6) help maintain energy levels and promote joint, brain, heart and vascular health, plus support healthy skin, hair and nails.

Keep your heart healthy
The statistics are frightening:

- Heart disease is the number one killer of both men and women in the United States and most of the western countries.
- Every 20 seconds, someone in the United States has a heart attack.
- One in four Americans has some form of heart disease.
- Every 34 seconds someone in the United States dies of heart disease.

Heart disease takes more lives than the next seven leading causes of death combined.

Processed food laden with hydrogenated oils and too many refined sugars are a huge contributing factor to the soaring numbers of heart problems in the West. To make your diet heart-healthy, eat more servings of fresh fruits and vegetables. Start your day with stewed apples or pears, include soaked blanched almonds in your diet, dress your veggies with fresh lime juice, and eat heart-friendly spices such as fresh-ground black pepper and turmeric (a powerful antioxidant). Choose fresh foods over processed foods or leftovers, light foods over rich, deep-fried ones, and warm, cooked foods over cold, heavy foods. Flax seeds provide excellent nutritional support for the heart. One spoon of apple cider vinegar diluted in some apple juice or water taken first thing in the morning helps to reduce cholesterol, which has been implicated in plaque build-up.

Get proper sleep

Sleep is just as important as diet in maintaining good health. Practice good bedtime habits; favor restful, calming activities an hour before bedtime to help the mind to disconnect from the senses. Keep your bedroom simple and clear of distractions such as television, computers, and other work related material. Maintain a temperature that's comfortable. Stay away from stimulants in the afternoon and evening. Go to bed before 10 p.m. The sleep before midnight is twice as effective as sleep after midnight. Studies link lack of sleep to blood pressure problems, depression and a multitude of health problems.

Soothe away stress

According to Ayurveda, excess stress (i.e. any overload on the system) is a fundamental cause of health problems, especially for the heart, not just on a physical level, but also on the subtler, emotional level. Sleep is essential to dissolve accumulated stress, but research shows that the additional level of deep rest experienced in meditation may also be required. Ayurveda has long regarded meditation to be a vital part of natural health care. Scientific studies, particularly on Maharishi Mahesh Yogi's Transcendental Meditation technique, indicates that practicing meditation twice daily lowers blood pressure, reversing arterial blockage and enhancing resistance to all types of stress (See next chapter). Herbal supplements can nourish the mind and emotions. Traditional Ayurvedic herbs such as *Brahmi*, *Ashwagandha* and *Arjuna* are renowned for their positive influence on the mind and emotional heart.

Cultivate positivism

While warding off excess stress is essential to prevent the emotional heart from wasting away, actively seeking mental and emotional wellbeing can help the emotional heart flourish. Ayurveda talks about *ojas*, a refined substance produced by the body that maintains life (it's what causes people's faces to "radiate" good health). The subtlest by-product of good digestion, *ojas* coordinates all activities of mind and body and leads to bliss, contentment, vitality and longevity. The cultivation of positive attitudes and emotions increases *ojas*. Ayurveda calls these behavioral *rasayanas* (tonics). Spend time everyday on those activities that give you contentment and happiness. Listen to soothing or uplifting music, enjoy serene and natural beauty, and use aromatherapy scents suited to your own body type and sip relaxing herbal teas. Always maintain a positive attitude and avoid situations that distress or anger you.

Regularly cleanse toxins from your physiology

Ayurveda recommends a program of internal cleansing known as *Pancha Karma* (literally, "five actions") with every change of season to help your body flush out accumulated toxins. These specialized treatment modalities are designed to remove accumulated toxins from the physiology using, amongst other things, oil and steam therapies. This has to be done under the expert supervision of a trained Ayurvedic doctor or technician. On a daily basis, you can help remove or reduce *ama* by drinking two cups of warm (boiled) water as soon as you wake up. This will clear out your stomach from any accumulated *ama* left over from improperly digested foods and give your digestive system a clean start for the day. Sipping hot or warm boiled water regularly throughout the day can also help the body digest *ama* (but don't overdo it!). The temperature should be according to your body type and

147

preference. Those with *pitta* constitutions, for example, will not be able to handle it too hot, whereas *vata* and *kapha* types can take it hot. I also recommend those with a propensity for high cholesterol to take one tablespoon of apple cider vinegar in a bit of water before breakfast. Apart from being the most natural and effective way to control cholesterol, apple cider vinegar will aid digestion and liver function. Ancient texts suggest taking half a teaspoon of raw honey after the vinegar. Only apple cider vinegar should be used as other vinegars contain different acids.

Go to bed by 10 p.m. to help the body cleanse itself during the natural purification time. Eat a lighter diet high in fiber and antioxidants from fruits, vegetables, whole grains and nuts. Avoid drugs, alcohol and smoking.

Mental *ama* can be minimized by avoiding negative input— such as violent TV shows, cinema and computer games—taken in through the senses. Avoid doubt and criticism of self and others. As some negativity is hard to avoid in modern life, I have found that meditation is the best possible way to wash away any residual mental *ama* that you may have picked up during your daily activity. At the same time it promotes inner happiness and mental and physical balance. If you enjoy taking a shower and feeling good and clean afterwards, you can imagine how meditation is like taking a shower on the inside. Once you get accustomed to feeling clean, blissful and peaceful inside, regular meditation will become as easy to practice as taking your morning shower.

⊙⊙⊙

Other views on health and back
According to traditional Chinese medicine, as we age the liver loses its capacity to perform or may become overheated. As a result the lower back literally "dries out" and the subtle force that maintains a correct posture

diminishes. Certainly it is not uncommon for poor liver function to go hand in hand with the loss of the lumbar curve. In this approach, the back problem is treated by healing the liver.

On the other hand many New Age healers say that back problems are all in the mind. If you have lower back pain it is because you have money worries and so the solution is to deal with the mental condition. As in the old story of the chicken and the egg, which one comes first— the physical condition or the mental condition—the liver problem or losing the sacrum–lumbar curve?

In truth, all these problems may be connected to back complaints and so one may conclude that the real root of the problem is much deeper and related to the subtle blueprint we have created for our bodies through the effect of our past actions (karma). Thus the best approach would be to attend to all the symptoms starting from their root. The psychological and mental stresses may be addressed by the practice of meditation. The drying-out or collapsing lumbar region can be helped by the practice of *MYOBack,* which will improve the nerve connection to the liver. And finally the health of the liver can be improved using traditional herbal medicines (Chinese, Ayurvedic or otherwise) and other procedures that may improve its performance.

LIVER CLEANSE

The liver, the body's purification system
In the human physiology, the liver is the organ chiefly responsible for filtering out toxins. The liver is full of tubes (bile ducts) that deliver the bile via the common bile duct to the gallbladder, which acts as a storage reservoir. If not looked after properly, over time, the liver can get clogged up just as any kind of filter can, resulting in an accumulation of sludge and debris that harbors unfriendly

149

bacteria and toxins. Stone-like formations can grow in the bile ducts that inhibit the liver and literally create a backup in the system much like a blocked drain can. These stones can be green, black, brown, red, white or tan colored. Liver stones, being porous, can pick up bacteria, cysts, viruses and parasites that are passing through. In this way nests of infection are formed that can be passed into the rest of the body creating such things as stomach ulcers, intestinal bloating, allergies, hives, and pains in the arms shoulders and upper back.

These stones are also high in cholesterol. Being low in calcium, they do not show on normal X-ray scans. Removing these stones from the liver ducts can greatly enhance liver functioning, increase energy levels, improve digestion, dramatically reduce cholesterol, and eliminate a whole range of illnesses, including back pain.

How to remove liver stones

There is a natural procedure to remove liver stones that is suitable for most people. However, if you have renal problems or suspected large gallstones it is better to check with your doctor first before attempting this procedure. If you have any doubt, ask your doctor anyway.

Note: Although this is a simple and natural cleansing procedure, it should not be used more than once every two or three years.

Ingredients required

Epsom salts   4 tablespoons   (60 - 80 grams)
Olive oil (good quality, virgin)   Half a cup. 125 cc (light olive oil is easier to get down)
Fresh pink grapefruit   1 large or 2 small, enough to squeeze 2/3 to ¾ cup of juice,
A one-liter jar with lid to mix the oil/grapefruit juice.
An enema kit from the pharmacy.

NOTE: For at least two weeks before cleansing the liver you should drink two cups of hot boiled water as soon as you wake up and then one spoon of pure natural organic apple cider vinegar in some water some twenty minutes later.

Choose a day like a Saturday for the cleansing, as you should be able to rest the next day.
Take no medicines, vitamins or pills that you can do without on the day of the cleansing as they could interfere with the success of the procedure.
Eat a no-fat, light breakfast and lunch. No butter or milk. Vegetarian diet is ideal. This allows the bile to build up and develop pressure in the liver. Higher pressure pushes out more stones.

1. **2:00 PM:** Do not eat or drink after 2 o'clock. You will need the body to have completed digestion and be settled before you start.
2. Mix **4 FULL** tablespoons of Epsom salts (80 rams), in one quarter liter of boiled water. You can keep the drink at room temperature.
3. **6:00 PM:** Drink one cup (250cc.), of the Epsom salts drink. Drink a little fresh water or rinse your mouth afterwards. If the flavor is a problem, try a bit of sugar, jam, lemon juice or other flavors. Better to drink quickly.
4. **8:00 PM:** Drink another cup of Epsom salts. If you already had a strong laxative response to the 6:00 PM drink, cut back to ¾ of a cup from now on. You won't have eaten since two o'clock, but you won't feel hungry as your body is busy with the cleansing. Ideally, the laxative effect of the Epsom salt should work by 10:00 PM, but don't worry if it hasn't, just continue with the instructions below.

5. Get ready to be in bed at 10:00 PM sharp. <u>The timing is critical</u>, so observe these instructions rigorously to obtain the best results.
6. **9:45 PM:** Pour ½ cup (measured) of olive oil into the one liter jar. Squeeze the grapefruit by hand into the measuring cup. Remove the pulp with a fork. You should have at least ½ cup (up to ¾ cup is best). You may top up with lemon juice if a bit short. Add this to the olive oil. Close the jar tightly with the lid and shake hard until you get a milky emulsion (only fresh grapefruit juice does this).
7. **10:00 PM:** Drink the olive oil and grapefruit juice emulsion standing up and lie down immediately afterwards. This is very important to get good results. Lie on your right side holding your right knee to your chest for 2 minutes and then lie on your back for another 30 minutes. This is the critical time in which the emulsion must go up the main liver duct and into the liver through its "back door". Stay lying in bed and allow sleep to come. You may feel the stones coming out of the liver ducts as it squirts bile out. If, after half an hour, you feel some heaviness in the stomach, turn your right leg over to the left while lying on your back, twisting the lower part of your body over to the left.
8. **6:00 AM:** In order to eliminate the stones that have gone to the intestine, you can take Epsom salts at 6:00 AM and 8:00 AM, or do an enema at 7:00 AM.
9. **7:00 AM:** Instead of Epsom salts you could do an enema of one cup of strong coffee plus the remaining Epsom salts. Make sure the liquid is at body temperature before you apply it.
10. **10.00 AM:** Approximately three hours later, you can prepare three spoons of rice boiled in two liters or more of water. Salt and spice to taste. Boil slowly for 30 minutes and then simmer until the water is

reduced and becomes a little thick in consistency. Drink water as required and if you are hungry take some of the rice gruel.

11. **LUNCH:** Take a light lunch and slowly return to normal food. You should be fully recovered by supper.

The effect of the Epsom salts will make the elimination very watery and the liver stones will float in the water due to their high cholesterol content. It is good to observe what is eliminated to make sure of the success of the treatment. Green stones are the most common, but you may also see brown or other colors and also small white crystals from the thinner liver ducts.

One should feel the difference a few days after treatment but the benefit can wear off a bit once more liver stones come down from the middle ducts. The cleansing could be repeated if it has never been done before. In this case, it is recommended to leave at least four weeks between cleanses.

Once you have had a big discharge of multiple colored stones you may not need to cleanse your liver for a number of years. You don't need to repeat the cleansing if you only eliminate green stones.

After proper cleansing, the liver will take some time to recover its full capacity, but then digestion will improve dramatically.

How safe is this procedure?
Anyone that is healthy enough to take a laxative can do it. Renal problems should be resolved before attempting this procedure. The elimination of gallbladder stones could be uncomfortable and even painful, but you should feel okay by the morning. For best results it is good to take the Epsom salts once (as in steps 5&6) some three days before

the full cleansing (it's like using the pre-soak" setting at the carwash!).

You can continue to drink two cups of hot boiled water on awakening and then one spoon of apple cider vinegar in some water some 20 minutes later as it will keep your cholesterol levels down, aid digestion and clear the stomach at the start of each day.

Chapter 7

Transcendental Consciousness and Peak Experience

Maslow and Peak Experience

My whole life, I have been interested in pursuing the furthest boundaries of human knowledge. While I was working for IBM during the 1980s, I was fortunate to have the opportunity to participate in a number of personal development courses, many of which had been developed by NASA psychologists to prepare astronauts for the first missions to the moon. They had to be ready for experiences that were literately out of this world. Much of the course content was based on the work of Abraham Maslow in the field of positive psychology.

Maslow discovered that, apart from the "normal" states of awareness known as sleeping, dreaming and waking, the human nervous system is able to experience a higher level of consciousness he referred to as "Peak Experience" or "Being", which he identified as the pinnacle of human experience. According to his research, all human beings function according to a "pyramid of needs". He identified these as:

1. The need to **HAVE**
2. The need to **DO**
3. The need to **BE**

These are organized in a pyramid structure as follows:

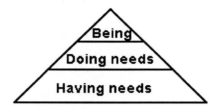

Fig. 77 Maslow's pyramid of needs

From an Ayurvedic point of view, these would correspond to Tamas, Rajas and Sattva. Maslow placed the first category – the need to HAVE, which deals with the body and the material world such as food shelter, etc – at the foot of the pyramid because they need the maximum amount of time and energy to achieve satisfaction (Tamas).

The second category – the need to DO, which deals with decision-making, problem solving and intellectual activity – he placed at the center of the pyramid, as they take considerably less energy to attain fulfillment (Rajas).

The third group – the need to BE, which deals with the subtler levels of existence such as Self-Realization or experience of pure Being – Maslow placed at the peak of the pyramid. At this level very little energy is required to fulfill needs (Sattva).

Each level of need creates a different form of perception and experience. In his work, Maslow described how people are able to move from one level to another. For example, at the top of the pyramid you could be engaged in some creative activity such as art or music, or a complex business deal, but when the time for dinner comes, a strong desire for food would emerge and you would drop a level into the "Need" category to satisfy your hunger. The impulses that motivate these desires and feelings are coming from a subconscious or subtle level, so we are never aware of how and when, or even why, they are generated. We can only be aware of the thoughts as they come to the surface of the mind. In any given day the average person human thinks 75,000 thoughts, however 95% of these are a repetition from the previous day and not necessarily particularly innovative. In other words, most of our minds are going round and round like a broken record repeating the same thoughts over and over again every day.

Maslow was particularly interested in the state of Peak Experience, and especially in the fact that creative and successful people seem to be most familiar with this state. He concluded that it is essential for human beings to regularly transcend the first two (lower) states of need *Having* and *Doing* in order to experience the higher state of *Being*, where desires get fulfilled effortlessly and where "full knowledge" is available. From his research, Maslow estimated that about one percent of the population can be classified as "successful" in their lives and that they frequently experience this higher state of Being, which he also referred to as Self Actualization. As result, these people feel more fulfilled and happy, enjoy more creative imagination, worry less, and experience more good luck. If removed from a successful position, they will quickly resume it due to a set of "fortunate" events.

Maslow's discovery of Peak Experience matches closely with the Vedic perspective of higher states of consciousness, which describes an inexhaustible supply of energy and intelligence that exists deep within the mind, in the area of experience that Maslow would call Being or Peak Experience. This is the source of all thinking and desires. The more we are able to have a clear connection with this level, the easier it is to fulfill our desires and, most importantly in the context of this book, maintain a good state of physical and mental health. This is what is meant by Self-Realization (or in Maslow's terms, Self-Actualization)—the ability the experience and operate from

157

the most expanded and unified level of consciousness, from which all the intelligence and energy that maintains not only our individual lives, but also that of the whole universe, originates.

Why do we feel pain?

From a Vedic perspective, pain arises, like all other difficulties and problems in life, when the mind and body are cut off from the natural flow of intelligence that supports, nourishes and maintains everything in the universe. We get out of harmony with Nature. Pain is a warning signal from the mind or body that something is going wrong and needs some attention. If we experience pain, including in our backs, then there is a good reason for it. It is not accidental. Ultimately, I am convinced that severe and chronic conditions are a cry from the inner Self, wanting to be awakened and discovered. In other words, there is a need for the experience of the state of Being or Self-Actualization that Maslow so eloquently described. Pain is the opposite of Peak Experience; Peak Experience is an antidote to pain.

It is through the accumulation of stresses of all kinds that the radiating light of Being gets distorted in a stressed-out man, and finally comes to the surface as negative feelings such as fear, anger, greed, compulsiveness, doubt and so on. This is why so many people are using medication to deal with the emotional pain their stresses are creating. The experience of the pure Bliss that exists at the level of Being generates a natural and free flowing positivity that doesn't depend on anything outside yourself. I believe the whole the purpose of human life is to move in the direction of more and more of this experience until it becomes permanent. This is what I would call Enlightenment. I have witnessed some miraculous recoveries when this path of evolution is taken.

Vedic knowledge also tells us that pain and suffering (including back pain) is connected to some past actions, either in this life or some previous existence (life is, after all, a continuous cycle of experience). These create deep stresses in our system. The principle of karma (action) is very simple and clearly defined in modern physics—for every action there is an equal and opposite reaction.

The universe is a myriad of interconnected energies. Every action we take, positive or negative, creates an effect in the whole universe. Think of how a stone thrown into a lake creates waves throughout the whole body of water. Each influence we create is eventually "bounced back" at us. Somewhere a running account is being taken of our actions; all bad debts have to be repaid and the benefits of all good investments enjoyed. From a health point of view, improper actions result in negative influences in our physiology that prevent it functioning properly, and so block the flow of natural intelligence. We have an alarm bell that tells us when something is going wrong: Pain.

It is impossible to intellectually understand all the millions of actions and reactions taking place in the universe that we are responsible for. Just to think about it alone would give us a headache. But we can understand the principle involved by a simple example such as when we eat some wrong food, we get a stomach ache.

The Vedic approach to this is not to worry about the problem but rather to solve it and thereby prevent it from happening again in the future. Ayurveda, as we have discussed, uses a multipronged approach to health that includes diet, exercise, herbal remedies, seasonal purifications and lifestyle in order to remove *ama* or toxins from the system and allow the free flow of natural energy and intelligence. It also recommends the use of deep meditation to contact the inner source of intelligence within the mind (Being). Not only does this open up the flow of intelligence into the mind and body, but also, according to

159

Vedic texts, it allows us to "roast the seeds" of our karma, whereby we can eliminate the results of past actions without having to experience the negative effects in our current lives. It enables us to firstly become a generator of more positive influences and less negative influences, and eventually to live in a state free from the effects of karma (and thus pain and suffering). This is the state of Enlightenment.

Finding Peak Experience

Maslow discovered Peak Experiences may occur at transition points between different states of consciousness, such as when you are falling asleep at night or waking up in the morning. At these times it is easy to experience clear understanding and creativity. (He kept a notebook next to his bed to write down the ideas he had at these times before they vanished from his mind). The problem is that these experiences are very brief and transitory.

After my initial experience with Maslow's programs, I set out to find ways to have Peak Experiences. I found I could effectively "forget" or transcend body awareness by doing progressive relaxation techniques or yoga exercises. But then I discovered that not being aware of the body caused the mind to become busier, thinking about all kinds of things. How could I stop the mind thinking and relax into pure silence or Being?

I remembered how settling the sound of waves was while lying on a beach on a warm summer evening. So, I decided to take my tape recorder and record different kinds of natural sounds to be used as a mind relaxation technique. I figured once I found the ideal natural sound, I could develop a technique that would allow me to go beyond body and mind. I also developed a form of "Water Yoga" where I would practice a combination of balanced breathing and swimming in the pool.

I passed on my discoveries in deep relaxation technique to my friends and family. But despite some soothing effects, the stresses of daily life began to pile up. My marriage ended in divorce and my ex-wife, Alicia, developed a number of serious health problems. It was obvious she was not getting enough benefit from my relaxation techniques. A doctor friend suggested we try meditation as he had recommended it to several of his patients with good results. I began searching the Yellow Pages for a meditation technique that would bring clear health benefits.

I attended many introductory presentations but always came away dissatisfied. The people involved never seemed to exhibit the good health that I was looking for. Then one day I was invited to a fundraising event organized by the Transcendental Meditation organization. I was pleasantly surprised to see a great number of people radiating good health and happiness, and the atmosphere in the room was very relaxed. The presentation on the scientific research on how the Transcendental Meditation (TM) technique can reverse the effects of ageing was also very impressive. With the help of my two daughters, we devised a plan for the whole family to learn. We discovered there was a family fee that would cover all of us. Once Alicia realized she could learn along with us at no extra cost, it was no problem getting her to attend the classes. She was far too curious to miss the opportunity.

The entire family benefited from practicing TM; not only did our health improve, but also our good fortune. Although Alicia continued to seek out other meditation practices, she soon realized there was nothing better than TM. One year later I was having problems finding her medical bills when I was preparing our tax returns. She had "forgotten" to go to the doctors. In my own case, I started to enjoy more and more bliss in my life. A supposedly "incurable" hearing problem in my left ear disappeared, and began to look and feel years younger than my age.

In just a few minutes practicing TM, I could experience what Maharishi Mahesh Yogi, the founder of the TM organization, calls Transcendental Consciousness, a state of restful "alertness" in which body and mind are completely relaxed and all that is left is the experience of timeless, eternal, pure Being. After years of searching I had found the way to experience Maslow's Peak Experience. Not only was the experience very satisfying and blissful, but as result of practicing the technique the stresses in my body seemed to fade away and I felt extremely relaxed and refreshed. Every time I practiced TM (twice a day for twenty minutes); I felt I was bringing something good into my life from the level of Being.

Tapping into the home of all knowledge.

After only three weeks of practicing TM, I started to "wake up" inside in the middle of the night. My body was still asleep but my mind was fully awake. It was a very blissful experience that lasted for many hours and repeated itself over several nights. It was as if I was able to "witness" the changing states of my awareness. Coming out of that state I could explore a new level of knowledge. It was as if my mind had no boundaries and I intuitively "knew" everything; like being the owner of a library of the whole universe, in which I could discover anything I wanted to know. Whenever I tried to consciously think about anything, my mind started to shrink back to the world of limitations. It was my first glimpse of the possibilities available when we regularly experience Being, or Peak Experience.

For thousands of years, the Vedic masters have talked about the existence of an unbounded field of consciousness that underlies all life in the universe and is the home of all knowledge, and which is accessible at the deepest levels of human awareness once the mind is operating at full potential. Modern day quantum physics describes a similar state known as the Unified Field, which is the origin of all the physical and energy forces in creation. Everything emerges from and returns to that state of existence.

Imagine how the world would be if all of us had access to such knowledge and such healing power.

Imagine a world free of pain, problems and suffering where everyone had use of their full potential to create success and happiness in their lives.

Scientists tell us we only use 5-10 % of our mental potential. Imagine if we used 100 %.

Chapter 8
The Grace of God

When good fortune smiles on us

When I was thirteen, I decided I wanted to visit my relatives on the island of Chiloe in southern Chile. I had never been on a plane before and I was excited about flying on a Douglas DC3, which I had heard so much about. I booked a seat without even thinking about how I would pay for it. When my mother broke the news that there was no money for my dream vacation, I didn't feel worried at all. I felt completely confident the money would somehow turn up for a plane ticket (I didn't even entertain the possibility of traveling by bus). Next thing I knew, all kinds of odd jobs were offered to me and at the end of three weeks I had half the money I needed. Then, right on the deadline for paying for the ticket, out of nowhere someone showed up to buy an antique piece (an old Spanish gun) that I had been trying to sell for almost a year. The price paid was exactly what I needed to pay the balance on my ticket.

While I was in Chiloe, I was able to earn enough money from helping on my relative's farms to pay for all my daily expenses. I never asked for money, it just came when I needed it. My cousin, Walter, couldn't believe my "good luck".

On the way home to Valdivia, I wanted to break my journey to visit the famous beauty spots in Puerto Montt, but I didn't have enough funds to pay for the change of ticket. Walter was convinced my "good luck" had run out. My plane had a scheduled stop in Puerto Montt before continuing to Valdivia, but without a change of ticket I couldn't leave the plane. After a long delay at Puerto Montt airport, however, the air stewardess informed me there was bad weather in Valdivia and, as I was the only passenger disembarking there, the plane was not going to land there. Imagine my surprise when they offered to put me up at a hotel in Puerto Montt for two days so I could catch the next flight to Valdivia. Walter couldn't believe my "luck" when I wrote to him to tell him about it.

At different times in our live, we all experience these strokes of easy good fortune, when everything seems to "just work out fine", without any effort our part. These are usually the most memorable times in our lives, when the Grace of God shines down upon us.

Maslow found that one percent of the population live in a state of awareness or consciousness that he called peak experience or Being. He also found that these people have constant good fortune which he attributed to that high level of consciousness. The question is then how to get to that high state of awareness.

The following is a quote from Maharishi Mahesh Yogi speaking at a course in Mergantheim, Germany, on 29 December, 1964, and transcribed in the book *Thirty Years Around the World; Dawn of the Age of Enlightenment.*

> "[The] Grace of God is all-pervading. It's always present. It's not that it comes; it is that we begin to make use of it. . . . There is nothing new that is to come; it has already come. It has not started with us as long as we have not started with it. The grace of God, the blessing of God, help from

God, doesn't come from anywhere. It is already there.

"Just like the air, it's already there. Now it is up to us to breathe it or not to breathe it. If we don't breathe, we begin to suffer. If we breathe, we begin to be normal.

"Like the air, the grace of God is available to us. It's permeating every fiber of our being and the being of the entire universe. Only, that which is the all-pervading grace of God is never isolated as an individual entity. It is just there. That which is to be all-pervading is not isolated, not bound, and that which is not bound is finer than the finest existence in creation. When we take our attention to that Being, finer than the finest, then we establish ourselves on the level of God's grace. Immediately we just enjoy. If we don't take ourselves to the level of God's grace, to that level of the finer than the finest, then remaining in the gross we don't have it.

"That is the story of the grace of God. He is said to be all-merciful . . . all-mercifully He has spread His grace much before we could want it. Much before the need could arise, it is there available for us.

"Through diving during meditation, we bring our attention, our conscious mind, to that level of grace, and we get filled with it completely. . . We associate ourselves fully with that grace and then enjoy. That is why this is the merciful nature of the Almighty. Very compassionately, very lovingly, He has spread His grace for us. Any time we can take our attention to that level, and we begin to own it. It's a matter of owning the grace of God. From His side He is available. From our side, as long as we hesitate to accept it, we hesitate to accept it. We get our-selves to that level, and it's already there.

"The Grace of God is like a full lake, a big lake full of water. Now, the water is there. Any farmer can take the water to his field. If the pipeline is not connected up to the level of water, the water remains.

"Water is just full, ready to flow. But it will not flow of its own accord. If the connection is made, it will naturally flow. If the connection is not made, it won't flow . . . and any man is free to make the connection from his field to the level of water. But if one doesn't make the connection, the water remains full.

"Just like the fullness of water in a lake or ocean, the grace of God is full. Those who make a connection, who draw the pipeline through Transcendental Meditation, to them it flows....Of itself it cannot flow."

Ritam Bhara Pragya

In my first year of university I was studying for the end of year examinations with a close friend of mine named Alfredo Puelma. We had made an arrangement throughout the year by which at least one of us would attend every lecture. That way, between us, we would end up with a full set of notes.

At three o'clock one morning, as we were preparing for the physics examination, we discovered that neither of us had a complete set of notes for one of the most important subjects. Being so late at night, we couldn't start calling our other friends on the phone, so we decided to grab some much needed sleep and deal with it in the morning. Four hours later, to my surprise, I woke up with all the points we needed flashing through my brain. I shook Alfredo awake and proceeded to give him a detailed lecture on the missing subject, including all the necessary formulas and deductions. I had no idea where it all came from, and it was hard to convince Alfredo that it was true, but when we checked with our friends that day, everything was accurate.

There is a level of creation in which everything exists in dormant form. This is a timeless, eternal field, where past, present and future coexist in a virtual state. In Vedic terms, this is known as *Purana*. Within *Purana* is the memory *(Smriti)* of every possible thing in creation. Between that silent, unmanifested and unbounded level of creation and the manifested or physical world we live in and appreciate through our senses, lies a thin layer like an onion skin where all possibilities begin to manifest. Known in Vedic terms as *Ritam Bhara Pragya*, this is the home of all knowledge. When we experience the level of *Ritam Bhara Pragya* within our own consciousness, the intellect, which is the more superficial level of the mind, is no longer involved and we enjoy the bliss of the great, unbounded cosmic mind. Here, everything is known with absolute certainty and stunning precision. When the young Mozart with almost no classical training produced his stunning musical masterpieces as if coming from nowhere, it was from this level that he was working. Here the individual mind merges with the omniscience of the Creator. It is like tapping into the universal cosmic computer from which all knowledge comes. It is the place from which the Grace of God emerges. It is also the level of awareness from where all Vedic knowledge (including that used in the *MYOBack* technique) spontaneously arises.

When Maslow talked about reaching the level of "real" creativity that exists at the peak of human experience, he was referring to this level of *Ritam Bhara Pragya* or the Grace of God. He understood very well the power of this experience, but he had no way of reaching it at will.

For thousands of year, since time immemorial, the Vedic masters of India have known the way to reach Peak Experience from whence the Grace of God shines bright. This is the Transcendental Meditation technique, most recently revived by His Holiness Maharishi Mahesh Yogi and made available to people throughout the world as a means to remove pain and suffering and create peace, health and harmony in everyone's lives. Generation after generation, great sages and enlightened saints from all religious and cultural traditions have demonstrated in their lives, the power of living in the Grace of God. That is why they are remembered and revered so much.

The fulfillment and happiness they achieved is now available to everyone, through the Grace of God and the wise teachers of the Vedic tradition.

Magical thinking

Maslow's research found that people frequenting or living high state of awareness or so called "peak experience" seem to have the ability to be in tune with nature and the surrounding environment. Like in the chicken and egg riddle it is hard to say how lucky events happen. Is it that the person can alter events or is the desire an anticipation of something that is perceived through intuition?

As a young child my close friend and I believed we had magical powers that could manifest any wish we made. On my twelfth birthday (December 26th) I told my friend I wanted to see a White Christmas like the ones we had seen on Christmas cards from friends in Europe and North America. That morning I announced I wanted to see everything—roofs, gardens and streets— covered in snow. I wanted to see my friends making snowmen and throwing snowballs. There was no doubt in my innocent child's mind that this was possible, even though where we lived in southern Chile we had never seen snow and we were well into the southern hemisphere's summer.

After lunch, my mother sent us to play in the rumpus room on the top floor of our house. I had completely forgotten about the White Christmas, when dark clouds began approaching overhead and soon a loud noise began to rattle the roof. It was a huge hailstorm! It didn't take long for everything to be covered in a massive layer of white. Cars couldn't move and everything was brought to a standstill. Our neighbors had to shovel the hailstones from their roofs for fear they would collapse under the weight! My friend freaked out. He was convinced we had produced the hailstorm and were powerless to stop it. As soon as the storm stopped all the kids ran out to play in the snow, make snowmen and throw snowballs to each other.

Is it possible we all have these magical powers to manifest or line up our desires with the oncoming events? Can we learn to live in tune with Mother Nature? I believe so and I agree with Maslow's findings.

The Grace of God and fulfillment of desires.

Once you are in touch with that level of the simplest state of awareness that Maslow described as Peak Experience, I believe you are in touch with the most powerful level of creation, from where any desire can be granted in the most gracious way. That is why we refer to it as "Mother Nature". A mother cannot refuse any request from her children.

The kind of language that Mother Nature understands is very simple and direct. If you want money, you may find a penny on the footpath and your desire "technically" is fulfilled, but probably not to the extent you wanted! So you need to be very precise and clear in the formulation of your desire.

When you reach that level of the simplest state of awareness or transcendental consciousness, a result of regular meditation, you become in tune with the Grace of God and your desires can be automatically be fulfilled. When the mind is relaxed and settled and thinking is merely a faint impulse, communication is possible with the most powerful and "loving" energy of the Creator. It is not possible to have any negative or harmful thoughts at this level. All you need to do is be absolutely precise about your desire and place your trust at the feet of God. Surrender without any force or pressure and let yourself "transcend" the desire. Only your doubts will stop you from fulfilling your desires. Once you have surrendered in total trust and without doubts, Nature will do what is right for you in silence and without any fuss.

I was once working in Sydney on an engineering project for IBM. One day, on my lunch break, I visited several automatic teller machines to get some cash to pay some urgent bills. I took out the maximum amount allowed for one day. That night I had to work late and I needed some extra cash to buy supper and gas for my car. I tried several teller machines hoping to get $60.00, but all of them refused me because I had already withdrawn the maximum amount. I went back to work thinking I would have to use my credit card instead and forgot the issue.

At around 8:00 PM my coworkers and I decided to break for dinner. The front doors of the building were closed for the day, so we had to exit through the lower parking level of a shopping mall. As we were walking through the car park, for some reason I drifted over to the right where I found a roll of three $20.00 notes lying on the ground. Nature had fulfilled my desire with stunning precision.

Although this is a small example of how precise fulfillment of desires can be, the mechanics are the same whether it is $60 or $6 million. And remember, Mother Nature has an inexhaustible supply of energy and intelligence at her disposal. All that is required is the regular access to the finest level of human awareness. The ancient Vedic masters knew how to gain access to this field of infinite intelligence within their own consciousness and thus they were able to cognize the finest levels of functioning of the laws of nature. This is from where the entire body of Vedic wisdom emerged. It was not learned or invented but realized at the deepest level of human consciousness.

Fortunately today, through the technique of Transcendental Meditation the stresses and strains that block access to this state of functioning are easily removed. Everyone now has the opportunity to tap into the finest levels of God's creation and fulfill their natural desire for peace, happiness and good health.

This is the real path to a life of fulfillment, free from pain and suffering.

Chapter 9
Life and Transformation

The miracle of life and transformation

There is no definite beginning or end to life. It is constantly creating and recreating itself, over and over again, from seed to flower to seed to flower, and so on. Behind it all is an incredibly intelligent master plan responsible for creating and managing infinite possibilities. The human body is no different from any other part of Nature. What we imagine to be "solid" bodies are actually ever-flowing streams of atoms and molecules that constantly emerge, return to, and reemerge from a field of infinite potential energy. Because there is a supreme intelligence behind the whole process, amazingly, despite all this change going on, we manage to retain a sense of individuality.

Mostly, we assume our bodies have a definite beginning and are moving inexorably toward a definite end. This is actually a mistake based on the lack of awareness of our full potential (as in Self-Realization or Peak Experience). If every minute of our lives some kind of genesis is going on and we are creating and recreating our physical structure over and over again, then it is never too late to begin creating the perfect body we really want, that is free from pain and problems.

Every breath we take is an act of creation. Think about what happens to a single oxygen atom as we breathe it in. Within a few thousandths of a second it passes through the lungs and attaches itself to the hemoglobin inside the red blood cells. In an instant, a remarkable transformation occurs. The blood cell changes color, from the dark blue caused by oxygen starved hemoglobin, to the bright red of oxygen-rich hemoglobin. A stray atom of air has suddenly become part of our body. It has crossed an invisible boundary from inert matter to a living being. In another sixty seconds that same oxygen atom will make a complete circuit of our body via the bloodstream (only fifteen seconds if you are exercising vigorously). In that time, about half of the body's new oxygen will exit the blood to turn into a kidney cell, part of a muscle, a neuron, or any other tissue. The atom will remain anywhere from a few minutes to a year, performing any function our body requires. This oxygen atom might become part of a happy thought by joining a neurotransmitter, or it might send a shiver of fear through your body by becoming part of a molecule of adrenaline. It could feed a brain cell with glucose or sacrifice itself to protect the body as part of a white blood cell fighting invading bacteria. This is how the river of life moves along with utmost fluidity and stunning intelligence and creativity.

Obviously, our responsibility to maintain good health is a very creative one. We have to manage a project that is equivalent to building a new universe every day. With every single breath, we expose around five trillion red blood corpuscles to the air. Each corpuscle contains 280 million molecules of hemoglobin. Each molecule of hemoglobin can pick up and transport eight atoms of oxygen. If you think of each oxygen atom as a new building block in your body, then with a single breath we are delivering 10 to 15 X 10 to the power of 21 (or 15,000,000,000,000,000,000,000) new "bricks" to various

176

construction sites around our body. According to the Divine Plan, each brick is placed with exact precision according to the intelligent blueprint contained within our DNA. Not a single new brick will disrupt the position of an old one. The old gives way to the new as smoothly and effortlessly as a river flows.

The only reason we are not functioning "perfectly" in a healthy manner, the only reason we experience pain and suffering, is because we disrupt this natural flow of intelligence by making mistakes such as eating wrong food, drinking impure water, breathing contaminated air, not doing the right exercises, or feeding ourselves unhealthy sensory input via TV, movies, and video games. In other words, our lives get out of tune with Natural Law. Our actions create wrong *karma,* which manifest as physical or emotional stresses. These, in turn, inhibit the natural flow of intelligence and the availability of Peak Experience. And so we come to believe that we are imperfect and limited. We engender destructive illusions such as "life is suffering", "life is difficult", and so on.

Why do we do this? Ultimately it is a matter of free will and where we put our attention. We choose to send signals to our bodies that repeat the same old beliefs, the same old fears and wishes, the same old habits of yesterday and the day before. So we end up stuck with the same old body.

Handling life as a whole
The new bricks that enter our body do not just fall into place; they are precisely positioned by cosmic intelligence that knows exactly how to build your heart, kidneys, skin, enzymes, hormones, DNA, and everything else. This intelligence is literally infinite, and yet available for our use in its entirety, at all times. For the most part, we take the boundless creativity of this quantum storehouse of energy and contain it with narrow beams of attention. Any thought

177

we have is a beam of focused energy sent out from our quantum self. Each thought has the ability to create a result in any direction in which we focus our attention. Where we put our attention grows more strongly in our lives. It takes only a few of these narrow beams of focused energy, or thoughts, to make life a little longer or a little better (or, if we so wish, a little shorter and a lot worse). For example, we can add, on average, five years to our lives by deciding to quit smoking. Or a few more years by losing excess weight, switching to healthy food, or taking regular exercise.

But these narrow beams of focused attention are limited. They will not make you perfectly healthy. In order to do this, we have to handle our infinitely complex quantum mechanical lives as a whole. Fortunately, the way to do this is surprisingly less complex than we would imagine. This gigantically complex project of creating ourselves day by day can be broken down into just a few processes. Let's review them:

Eating is the creative act that selects the raw matter of the world that will be turned into you. To make sure this process proceeds correctly, you need only to know your body type and follow the diet that matches it. Consult an Ayurvedic doctor or trained Ayurvedic consultant on your body-type diet; let the information sink in by discussing it until you have absorbed the guiding principles. Now eat according to those principles, easily and comfortably.

Digestion and assimilation are the creative acts that turn the "bricks" of matter into living tissue. Your body's digestive fire (agni) handles both of these processes in perfectly coordination. Follow Ayurvedic advice and learn how your particular kind of body functions, and then respect your digestive fire by following this advice.

Elimination is the creative act that purifies the body, excreting undigested food and ridding the cells of toxins and other "old bricks." You can improve elimination by being regular in your daily routine, drinking plenty of water and having a good level of fiber content in your diet. You may also add the help of purifying herbs. A sattvic diet is also a great help, since it reduces to an absolute minimum the intake of impurities. If you can, incorporate seasonal Ayurvedic purifying treatments (panchakarma) into your annual routine, preferably three times a year, but at least once. This is the most powerful therapy for aiding elimination.

Breathing. Make sure you get to breathe clean air as much as possible, so that the airborne building blocks are of the best quality. The air near large masses of water will generally be purer and will contain more vitality (prana). As the basic rhythm of life that supports all other rhythms, breathing could be called the most creative act we perform each day. Correct breathing tunes our cells to the rhythms of nature, and the more natural and refined our breathing, the more in tune we become. Many Ayurvedic routines help to bring breathing back into balance. Exercise according to body type is good, as is the gentle form of Pranayama (yogic breathing exercises) for a few minutes each day. You can probably learn a type of Pranayama at your local yoga class.

Exercise stimulates the vitality of the body, maintains flexibility, enhances the distribution of oxygen, aids digestion and keeps the metabolic rate healthy.

Transcend. This is the most important one of all, and brings all the other processes under one heading. By taking the awareness to the home of intelligence deep within the mind (Peak Experience), it allows us to live in tune with the subtlest aspects of our mind and body. It automatically reconnects us with the natural intelligence that guides us all aspects of our lives. This is the most creative act of life. If you live in tune with your subtle body, all of your daily activities—breathing, eating, digesting, assimilating, and eliminating—will proceed more smoothly and effortlessly.

Learn a good meditation technique and practice it regularly. Personally, I highly recommend Maharishi's Transcendental Meditation technique.

Value your inner self above your material possessions such as your car or house. These are all temporary adjuncts to your life. You cannot take them with you as you progress and evolve in life.

If we follow these simple guidelines, our lives will remain in balance and run as effortlessly as the cycle of the seasons or the ocean tides.

The Ocean of Consciousness

We tend to think of ourselves as distinct individuals living alongside other, separate individuals and against a "backdrop" of the natural world. We don't understand how everything is interconnected and how our own actions and our own state of health affect others. Vedic sages looked at life through different eyes. A famous Vedic verse says, "It is our duty to the rest of mankind to be perfectly healthy, because we are ripples in the ocean of consciousness, and when we are sick, even a little, we disrupt cosmic harmony."

We are not isolated organisms in time and space, occupying six cubic feet of volume and lasting seven or eight decades. Rather, we are one cell in a vast cosmic body, entitled to all the privileges of our cosmic status, including bliss and perfect health. God gave us self-consciousness so we could realize this truth. As another Vedic verse declares, "The inner intelligence of the body is the ultimate and supreme genius in nature. It mirrors the wisdom of the cosmos."

At the subtlest level of Creation, there is no sharp boundary dividing you from the rest of the universe. Each of us is a balance between the finite and the infinite, localized form and unbounded potential. The same protons found at the heart of stars five billion years old, also take residence inside us. The neutrinos that streak through the earth in a few millionths of a second are part of us for a brief instant too. You are a flowing river of atoms and molecules collected from every corner of the cosmos. You are a projection of energy whose waves extend to the edges of the unbounded unified field. You are a part of a reservoir of intelligence that cannot ever be exhausted. The whole universe is a living, breathing, thinking organism of which we are an intimate part.

And the purpose of this huge cosmic display of infinite energy and possibilities is that we should live abundantly healthy and happy, free from pain and suffering.

Most important of all, we should ENJOY.

Chapter 10

Yoga and total health

Life should be lived in total harmony and integration. Talking about back pain as an isolated bone problem is incomplete without contemplating life as a whole.

One of the primary definitions of the word "Yoga" is "union". The objective of yoga is to attain total union or integration of body mind and spirit or Being. This state, where life is experienced in total integration is spoken of clearly in Ayurveda and also in Maslow's pyramidal representation of the stages of human consciousness.

Just as in Yoga, achieving full potential is the goal of Maslow. The difference is that he didn't have a method to get there, whereas for thousands of years the yogis of India have been developing the path to achieving integration or unity.

The Yogis of India practice asanas not just to keep a healthy spine but as in Maharishi's systematic teachings the objective is to provide the method to achieve full potential and integration in life. And one of the results of this practice is a very healthy spine.

It would be incomplete to talk about just back bones without looking at the totality and what is life as a whole.

The ultimate truth of life.

This world is populated by temporary citizens. The average person visits our planet for only seventy or eighty years, and yet most people seems to be living as if they will never leave or die; they waste their time on quantity and gratification of the senses and do not develop their full capacity to experience the quality of life in its most fulfilling sense. So many people spend their entire lives chasing imaginary and ephemeral goals that at the end of the day (or life), they have absolutely no real value or meaning for what rests ahead.

When it is too late to change, many find themselves feeling frustrated and empty as their life's accumulated glitter or wealth suddenly loses its value.

Our time and energy are our most valuable natural resources. It is our choice as to how to spend them. We can use them wisely or throw them away.

Do you want to live pain free, happily, and in good health? Believe it or not we have choice. The higher we live in Maslow "hierarchy of Being" or in the higher states of consciousness described by Maharishi, the more in tune we live with Mother Nature and the easier we will achieve our goals and desires.

The law of cause and effect is immutable. As we support life and nature, good luck supports us, as even Maslow's research implied.

If we have been suffering pain it is for some reason or karma and if the solution comes it is because we have passed that lesson and must move on. Establishing ourselves at the top of the pyramid or Being empowers us to spontaneously perform right action. Right action is free from negative consequences. The result is healthier and happier life in harmony with our surrounding environment.

God gives us freedom of choice. We don't have to suffer. No one is forcing us to be unhappy or in pain. Nothing is written in stone. There is no "have to" in life at all. We work, we pay our bills, we love, we fight, we do all the things we do in life because we choose to even though often we may feel as if we were the victims of some external influences.

So much stress is created by the mistaken belief that there is no choice, when in fact there is. The only "have to" in this life is that one day we have to die. Otherwise, we always have a choice. Of course there are consequences to our choices but it is important for us to know there is no "have to" involved.

Everything that happens to us in life happens exactly as it should happen it is a consequence of our own past actions (karma). We write the screenplay for the film that we star in. There is no one else to blame if things are painful or difficult. What we did in the past has created our current state of life. We made our choices and we cannot change them, so we must deal with what we have created.

However, we can change things for the future, starting right now by making new and better choices. We can free ourselves from pain. We can live a healthy life. We can live up to our full potential. It is our choice.

So much vital energy is wasted in creating stress in our lives and suffering the consequences. So much time and energy is wasted worrying about things. How many times, for example, have you spent hours exhausting yourself worrying about a problem, only to find that when out of exhaustion you relax, the solution comes to you? Wouldn't it be better to stop punishing ourselves wasting our valuable resources, solve the problem and get back to enjoying life? Shouldn't everything in life be so effortless? If we are using only five percent of our brain's capacity how can be claim to be awake? Wouldn't it be better to use the full 100%, so we can really wake up and appreciate the full value of life? Self-Realization, Enlightenment, Self-Awareness, Bliss and happiness, Nature's support or you may say good luck or living the Grace of God, Peak Experience, whatever you want to call it isn't this a worthwhile goal? Given freedom of choice, which we have, wouldn't we be crazy to choose anything else but the best? What is the best way to spend our valuable resources of time and energy?

There is plenty of evidence of enlightened civilizations having existed in the past, not only in India but also in the Americas, the Middle East, and all over the globe; times or places where people lived in perfect harmony with Natural Law, respected every aspect of God's creation, and, as a result, life was Bliss not only for the individual, but for society as a whole. I am convinced that with the current revival of Vedic knowledge, a new Golden Age is approaching in our time just like those in the past; a time when all people will be connected to the highest state of human consciousness, when everyone will live life to its fullest glory, when no one will suffer pain of any kind, and life on earth will become Heaven on Earth. With the knowledge we now have available, each of us can create this in our lives and in the life of our community. It is our choice.

I hope this book not only helps heal your pain but also sets you on the path to full realization and heavenly Bliss. I look forward to your good health, happiness and Enlightenment.

All Glory to Maharishi Mahesh Yogi for his tireless work in bringing this precious Vedic wisdom to our homes and hearts. All Glory to Guru Dev and the Masters of the Vedic Tradition whose only desire is everyone should enjoy Heaven on Earth.   Jai Guru Dev

Lightning Source UK Ltd.
Milton Keynes UK
05 May 2010
153743UK00001B/56/P